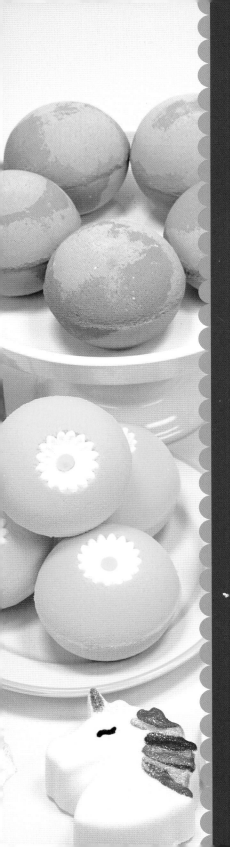
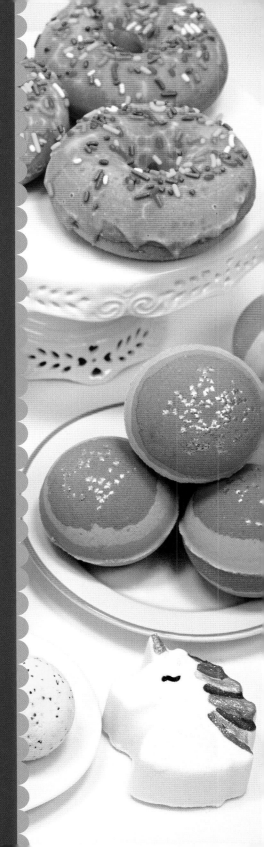

HOMEMADE
BATH
BOMBS
& MORE

Soothing Spa
Treatments
for
Luxurious
Self-Care
and
Bath-Time
Bliss

HEIDI KUNDIN

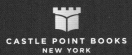

CASTLE POINT BOOKS
NEW YORK

For Mitch, for always supporting all of my crazy creative endeavors, and without whom none of this would have ever been possible (seriously!). For Sawyer, Sutton, and Simon for always being willing testers and participants in my crafty experiments. I love you guys with my whole heart! xoxo

. . . .

The Castle Point Books trademark is owned by Castle Point Publications, LLC.
Castle Point books are published and distributed by St. Martin's Press.

ISBN 978-1-250-26593-7 (hardcover)
ISBN 978-1-250-25308-8 (ebook)

Design by Hillary Caudle
Photography by Heidi Kundin

Our books may be purchased in bulk for promotional, educational, or business
use. Please contact your local bookseller or the Macmillan Corporate and
Premium Sales Department at 1-800-221-7945, extension 5442, or by email at
MacmillanSpecialMarkets@macmillan.com.

First Edition: February 2020

10 9 8 7 6 5 4 3 2 1

CONTENTS

::::::::::::::::::::::::::::

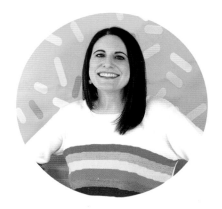

WELCOME

....

*B*ath bombs are an explosion of sensory bliss. Vibrant colors create pretty, fizzy pools of stress relief as heavenly scents soothe your mind and body. Rich, creamy bubbles nourish your skin and turn bath time into a lush at-home spa experience.

Bath bombs are one of my favorite ways to treat myself and enjoy self-care. That's why I'm so excited to share *Homemade Bath Bombs & More*! In the pages that follow, you'll find more than 75 easy recipes for bath bombs and other homemade bath and body products that are specially formulated to turn any day of the week into a spa day.

Do the often outrageous costs of store-bought products hold you back from indulging in regular bath bomb treatments? The DIY recipes in this book are just what you need! Not only are bath bombs a fun project for both beginning and advanced crafters, you also control what goes into your bath products, and you control the costs. Each product is made from naturally derived skin-pampering ingredients that are designed to leave your body feeling moisturized, rejuvenated, glowing.

And don't forget that the bath bombs and other bath products in this book make great homemade gifts too! Keep some on hand or design a thoughtful bath gift with a specific recipient in mind.

So, what are you waiting for? Let's add some luxurious self-care to bath time!

DIY BATH

BLISS

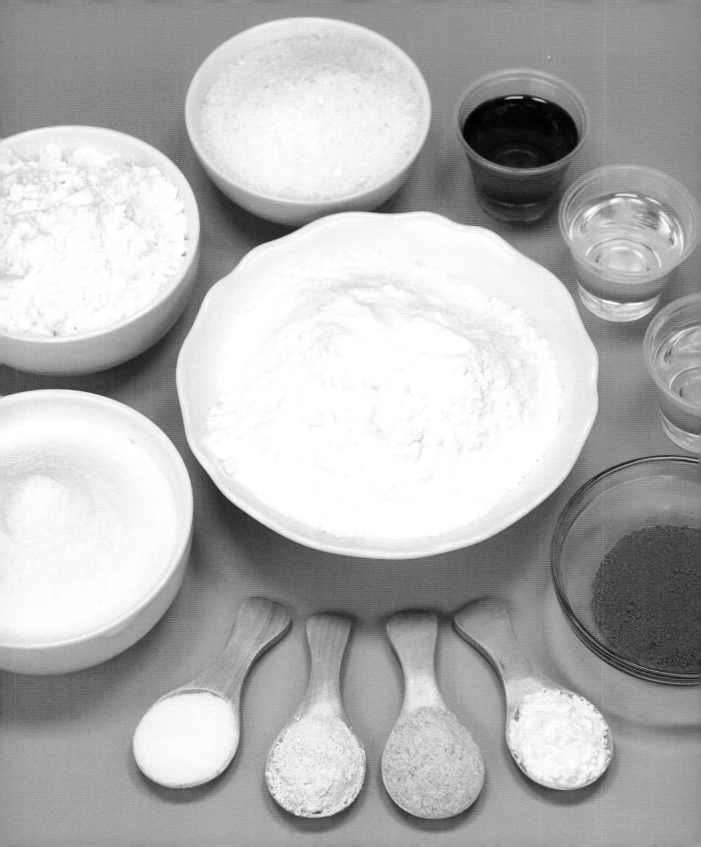

ABOUT THE INGREDIENTS

*B*eyond heavenly self-care, what exactly is packed into a bath bomb? The two primary ingredients in bath bombs are simply sodium bicarbonate (baking soda) and citric acid. When combined with water, these ingredients cause an acid-base chemical reaction that releases carbon dioxide and causes a fizzing effervescent reaction in the bathtub. Bath bombs may also contain surfactants to add bubbles, colorants to make things pretty, and oils and/or butters for extra nourishing skin and health benefits. Some of the most common ingredients can be found at your local grocery store; others are easily found through online retailers or at craft supply stores.

This book includes many different recipes for bath bombs, and the success of each recipe will largely depend upon the climate and conditions of your geographical location. High humidity, for example, might require you to use slightly less liquid than a recipe calls for, whereas drier conditions might require you to add a bit more moisture to your mixture. It is helpful to know the role that each ingredient plays in the recipe in order to understand bath bomb chemistry. This background will help you to determine the appropriate combination of ingredients that will provide you with the best bath bombs. A little learning will also help you feel comfortable with what you are bringing into your bath and shower. It may even inspire you to develop your own creative recipes!

Activated charcoal: This ultra-fine black powder is often used to color bath bombs. It is also known for its ability to deeply cleanse and exfoliate skin and to detoxify the body.

Arrowroot powder: This ingredient is used to harden bath bombs and remove excess moisture.

Baking soda (or sodium bicarbonate): The main ingredient in bath bomb recipes, baking soda softens water and leaves skin feeling smooth. Sodium bicarbonate is considered a "weak base"

and will cause a fizzy acid-base reaction when combined with water and citric acid, a "weak acid."

Butters: Butters add moisturizing properties to your bath bombs to make skin extra smooth and silky. Commonly used butters include avocado, cocoa, coffee, mango, and shea. ***Caution:*** *Bath bombs that contain butters may make your bathtub slippery.*

Citric acid: This naturally occurring weak acid is derived from citrus fruits. It is most often used at a 1:2 ratio along with baking soda to create a bath bomb's fizzing reaction. Citric acid also kills bacteria and helps leave the tub squeaky clean after your bath!

Clays: Used to help harden bath bombs, clays are also a natural detoxifier. The most commonly used clays for bath bombs are bentonite clay and white kaolin clay.

Cocamidopropyl betaine: This biodegradable organic chemical compound (derived from coconut) has exceptional foaming properties and produces lots of fluffy bubbles in your bathtub.

Cornstarch: As a dry "filler" ingredient, cornstarch is used to thicken other ingredients and to help harden bath bombs. Be careful not to overdo it, though, because too much cornstarch in your recipe can reduce the intensity of the fizzing reaction.

Cosmetic glitter: Specifically formulated for skin contact, cosmetic-grade glitter adds sparkle and shimmer to bath bombs.

Essential oils & fragrance oils: Essential oils are naturally distilled oils that can add both fragrance and purported health benefits to your bath bombs. Synthetic fragrance oils are generally far less expensive than essential oils and are available in an abundance of scents.

Isopropyl alcohol: At 90 percent concentration or higher, isopropyl alcohol can be used as a binder for bath bombs. It is also a key ingredient for making mica "paint" to add details to your bath bombs.

Micas: These natural pigment powders are derived from crushed minerals and used to add color to bath bombs. Micas are cosmetic-safe and are available in shimmery, pearl, or matte finishes.

Milk powder: Powdered milks contain fats and proteins that exfoliate and moisturize skin and can help with eczema and psoriasis. Buttermilk powder can also be used in place of sodium lauryl sulfoacetate (see below) to create gentle foam and bubbles in bath bombs.

Oatmeal: Ground into fine colloidal oat powder, oatmeal is a great addition to bath bombs and helps to soothe dry and itchy skin.

Oils: Used to add moisture to the bath bomb recipe, oils bind the mixture together. All oils have moisturizing properties that hydrate and soften skin, and different varieties of oil also lend various additional benefits. Coconut oil, for example, is known for its antiaging properties. The most popular oils to use in bath bombs are sweet almond, avocado, coconut, grapeseed, and jojoba. ***Caution:*** *Bath bombs that contain oils may make your bathtub slippery.*

Polysorbate 80: This vegetable-based emulsifier helps oil-based ingredients disperse more evenly in the bath water. It is also used to prevent mica colorants from leaving a ring around the bathtub.

Salts: Reported to soothe sore muscles and dry skin, magnesium-rich Epsom salt is a common bath bomb ingredient. Sea salt and pink Himalayan salt are also frequently used in bath bomb recipes due to their reputed detoxifying properties. Salts attract water and can occasionally start the fizzing reaction prematurely, so they should be included in minimal to moderate amounts only. Grinding salts to a fine powder will produce the best results and smoothest finish on your bath bombs.

Sodium lauryl sulfoacetate (SLSA): When added to bath bombs, SLSA creates thick and luxurious foamy bubbles during the fizzing process. SLSA is naturally derived from coconut and palm oils and is safe for sensitive skin.

Vegetable glycerin: Often added to cosmetics to better combine oil- and water-based ingredients, vegetable glycerin is known to moisturize skin and leave it feeling supple and hydrated.

Witch hazel: This ingredient is the most commonly used liquid binder for bath bombs. A scant amount is used to bring the mixture to the proper consistency and help the ingredients adhere together.

ABOUT BATH BOMB MOLDS

Traditional bath bomb molds are available in a wide variety of styles and materials. With the recent rise in popularity of custom 3D-printed bath bomb molds, the only limit is your imagination! Create unique bath bombs in all kinds of creative shapes and themes.

Round ball molds: Two-piece ball-shaped bath bomb molds are widely available in stainless steel, aluminum, and plastic varieties. Metal molds are generally more durable and easier to release than their plastic counterparts.

Metal molds: Metal bath bomb molds come in numerous shapes and sizes, and they make an excellent molding choice due to their stability and ease of use.

Hard plastic molds: Hard plastic molds are terrific for molding fun novelty-shaped bath bombs. The rigid surface of the hard plastic allows you to firmly pack the bath bomb mixture as required, and the molds tend to release with relative ease. Plastic molds that are designed for bath bombs and soaps are the best, but molds for chocolate-covered sandwich cookies are another great option.

Candy molds: Hard plastic candy molds can also be used to make bath bombs. However, due to their shallowness, they are usually best for making embellishments or colorful embeds to place inside of larger bath bombs.

Three-piece plastic molds: Three-piece, 3D-printed plastic molds are quickly gaining popularity thanks to their ease of use and limitless design possibilities. Avoid washing these molds in hot water as the plastic can warp or melt easily under high heat.

Silicone molds: Silicone molds come in an endless variety of shapes and sizes, so it's unfortunate that they aren't the most ideal molds for making bath bombs. The flexibility of silicone makes it challenging to properly pack and mold the bath bomb mixture, but success can be found with practice and patience.

Household items: Many household items can also be used to mold bath bombs. Paper cups, small bowls, cupcake pans, mooncake molds, cookie presses, and other gadgets can all be used for making bath bombs. Use your imagination and start putting some unique household items to the bath bomb test!

Tip: For a detailed list of the bath bomb molds that were used in this book and their suppliers, visit happinessishomemade.com/bath-bomb-molds

ABOUT ADDITIONAL SUPPLIES

Making bath bombs requires just a few basic supplies, but it's important to prepare your workstation ahead of time. Bath bomb recipes are time-sensitive, starting to dry out quickly after mixing, so it's necessary to have all your supplies in place before you get started.

Mixing bowls & spoons: A large mixing bowl (approximately 4-quart size) will be needed for each color in the bath bomb recipe.

Measuring cups & spoons: Any traditional measuring utensils will do—no need to get fancy.

Tip: Keep two sets of measuring spoons at your workstation—one for dry ingredients and one for liquids—to speed up the measuring and mixing process.

Scale: Many of the recipes in this book are measured in US standard kitchen measurements; however, some call for a kitchen scale for more precise measurement and control of your ingredients.

Stand/hand mixer: A stand or hand mixer is incredibly helpful for quickly and thoroughly mixing ingredients but is not required. Good old-fashioned hand mixing works just as well with a little patience!

Gloves: Gloves are recommended for both sanitary and practical purposes. Citric acid can sting if it comes into contact with small cuts and scrapes, and some concentrated micas can stain your hands, so gloves are recommended to avoid any mishaps.

Mask: Mixing dry bath bomb ingredients can cause a cloud of fine particles in the air, so wearing a mask is highly advised to prevent inhalation of the ingredients.

Cyclomethicone: This synthetic silicone oil can be used to coat the inside of a bath bomb mold for easier release.

Drying trays & foam: Freshly unmolded bath bombs need to sit undisturbed for at least 12 hours while they dry and firm, so using a drying tray to move them from one location to another is a must. Line the tray with a thin layer of foam or padded material for flat bath bombs or foam egg crate material for round bath bombs.

HOW TO MAKE & MOLD BATH BOMBS

Each bath bomb recipe has its own unique combination of ingredients and measurements, but the basic mixing and molding process is always the same. Follow the foolproof step-by-step directions that start on page 11, and you'll be making awesome bath bombs in no time!

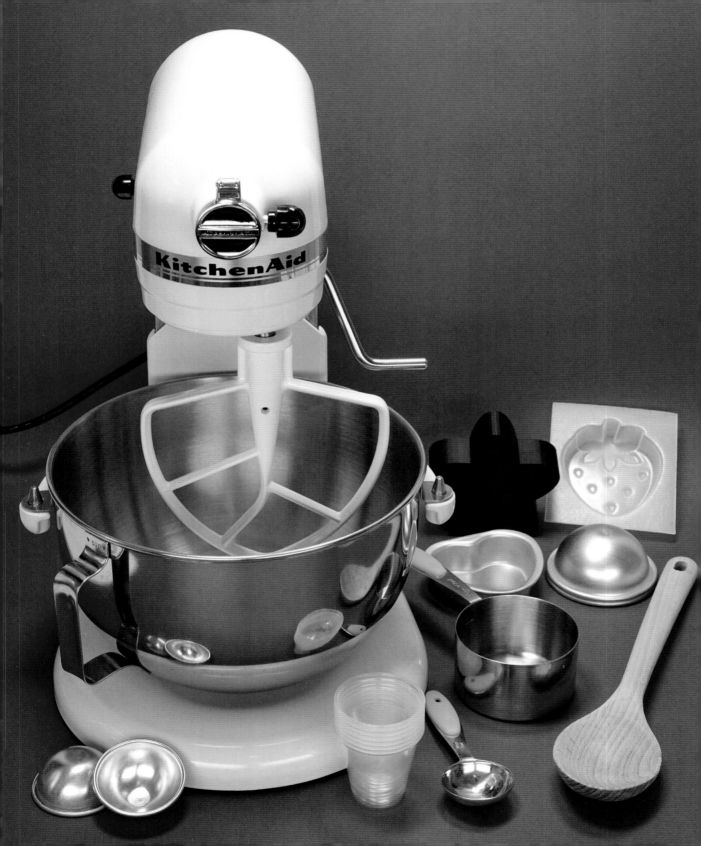

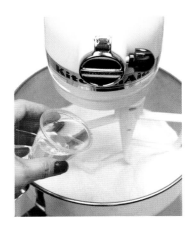 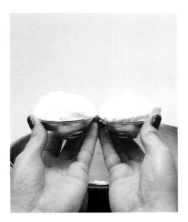 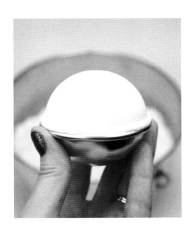

MAKING BASIC BATH BOMBS

1 · In a large bowl, sift the baking soda to remove any clumps. Sift the citric acid into a smaller bowl and set aside for later.

2 · Add the remaining dry ingredients to the baking soda bowl and mix well.

3 · In a small container, combine the oil and other liquid ingredients.

4 · Stirring constantly, slowly pour the liquids into the dry ingredients and mix until they are thoroughly combined. *(Note: Stir quickly to ensure that the fizzy mixture doesn't start to activate when you introduce the liquids!)* Make sure that all of the wet ingredients are evenly incorporated into the dry mixture for the proper texture and consistency.

5 · Slowly add the citric acid to the bath bomb mixture a little bit at a time, stirring constantly, until it is fully incorporated.

6 · Use your hands to test the moldability of the mixture. It should feel like damp sand and hold together when squeezed between your hands.

7 · If the mixture is not quite wet enough to mold, spritz two to three times with a spray bottle of witch hazel and mix well. Repeat as necessary.

MOLDING BATH BOMBS

· For traditional round ball molds, lightly pack the bath bomb mixture into both halves of the mold and generously overfill each side of the mold. Press the halves firmly together and brush away any excess.

· When unmolding round bath bombs, remove half of the mold at a time and allow the bottom half of the bath bomb to rest in the other half of the mold while the top half of the bath bomb dries. This step ensures that the bottoms of your bath bombs stay rounded and don't flatten out. Flip the mold to the opposite side of the bath bomb after an hour and then unmold completely after 2 hours. Allow to dry completely for 24–48 hours.

· For metal or hard plastic molds, use your fingers and palm of your hand to firmly pack the bath bomb mixture into the mold. Fill the mold to the top until it is packed completely full. Carefully release the bath bomb from the mold and allow to dry completely for 24–48 hours. Alternately, for more delicate and detailed molds, you may wish to allow the bath bombs to dry inside the molds and then release.

· For 3D-printed three-piece molds, place the bottom half of the mold inside the ring and very lightly pack the bottom layer. Loosely fill the rest of the mold with bath bomb mixture, overfilling just

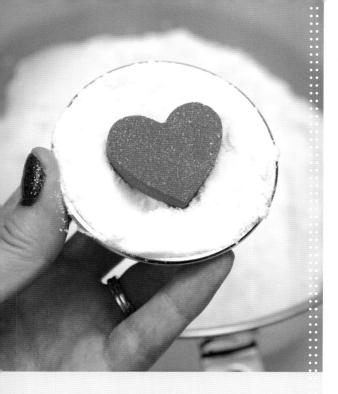

slightly, and press the top half of the mold firmly into the ring. Flip the mold over and press again from the opposite side. Slide the ring off of the mold, and carefully unmold the bath bomb. Allow to dry completely for 24–48 hours.

Tip: If you have difficulty unmolding your bath bombs, you may wish to coat the inside of the molds with a thin layer of cyclomethicone for easier release.

TIPS & TRICKS

• You can simply reuse the same mold to create each bath bomb from the recipe's mixture. Or you can purchase multiple molds to speed the process and include helpers.

• "Spray painting" is an easy way to add color to finished bath bombs. Mix together cosmetic mica powder and isopropyl alcohol in a fine-misting spray bottle and spray away. A 1:2 ratio of mica to alcohol usually works best.

• Save time by purchasing premade colored embeds from your favorite bath bomb supply sellers. You can even find rainbow-colored embeds that include all the colors of the rainbow in one embed.

• "Fairy duster" bottles of cosmetic glitter allow you to quickly and easily spray a fine mist of dry glitter on an entire batch of bath bombs in just a few seconds.

• Don't toss out crumbled or broken bath bombs! Repurpose them as fizzy bath powder and enjoy the same relaxing benefits in powdered form.

HOW TO MAKE EMBEDS

*B*ath bomb embeds can add an extra punch of color and fun to the center of your bath bombs.

1 · In a large bowl, sift together equal parts of baking soda and citric acid to remove any clumps. Add mica colorants or FDA-approved color additives (lakes or dyes) for an even stronger punch of color.

2 · In a spray bottle, mix together equal parts water and isopropyl alcohol. Spray the dry mixture several times, stirring quickly to avoid activating the mixture, until the mixture is a moldable consistency.

3 · Use mini ice cube trays or small hard plastic molds to mold the embeds. Allow to dry for 24–48 hours before using.

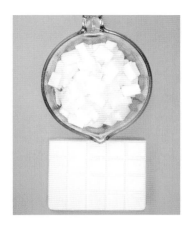
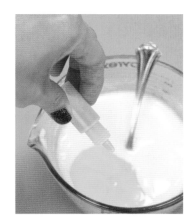
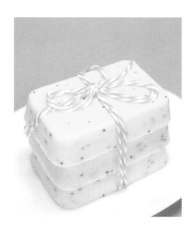

HOW TO DESIGN SOAP

*C*ustomizing your own soap has never been easier than this simple melt-and-pour process!

CUSTOMIZING MELT & POUR SOAP:

1 · Cut the soap base into approximately ½″ square cubes.

2 · Place the soap cubes into a microwave-safe measuring cup. Melt the soap in the microwave in 30-second increments, stirring well after each session to ensure that the soap is completely melted.

3 · Carefully stir in your desired soap colorant, fragrance, and any additional mix-ins.

4 · Pour the melted soap into the mold and spray the top of the soap with isopropyl alcohol to break the surface tension and remove any air bubbles.

5 · Allow to cool undisturbed for 60–90 minutes or until completely firm (time will depend on temperature and humidity).

6 · Unmold and enjoy!

TIPS & TRICKS

· When adding mix-ins to your melt-and-pour soap, make sure you're using a soap base that is labeled as "suspension." Suspension soap base will allow your mix-ins to disburse evenly throughout the soap; in nonsuspension base, the mix-ins will settle to the bottom of the mold.

· Red soap colorant has been known to slowly bleed into other colors in multicolored soaps. For example, the red colorant might eventually turn the adjacent white layer of your watermelon soap pink. Look for a red colorant that is labeled as "non-bleeding" to ensure crisp color lines with no bleed.

· Silicone molds work best for melt-and-pour soap making.

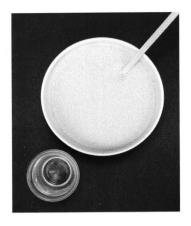 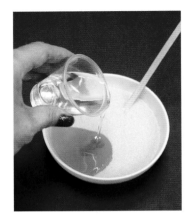 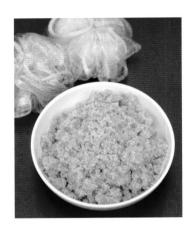

HOW TO MAKE SCRUBS

$\mathcal{S}$crubs leave your skin feeling silky smooth, and they are one of the quickest and easiest homemade bath and body products that you can make! Scrubs made from sugar are the most popular choice, but salt-based scrubs are also a trendy option. (Just be sure to avoid using salt scrubs on any areas with cuts or irritated skin—*ouch!*)

MAKING SUGAR SCRUB

1 · Pour sugar into a medium-sized bowl.

2 · Add powdered mica colorant to the sugar and stir until well combined.

Tip: The color of the scrub will be darker and more vibrant once the liquid ingredients have been added.

3 · Mix the oil and any additional liquid ingredients together and add to the dry ingredients. If you prefer a more liquid scrub, add more oil by the ½ teaspoon until you reach the desired consistency.

USING SUGAR SCRUB

1 · In the bath or shower, scoop up a small amount of sugar scrub and gently rub all over your hands, feet, and body (being careful to avoid delicate areas) for smooth, soft, and moisturized skin.

2 · Rinse well and pat skin dry with a soft towel. **Note:** *Use caution when using sugar scrubs in the bath and shower, as the oils can make the surface slippery!*

SWEET

LUXURY

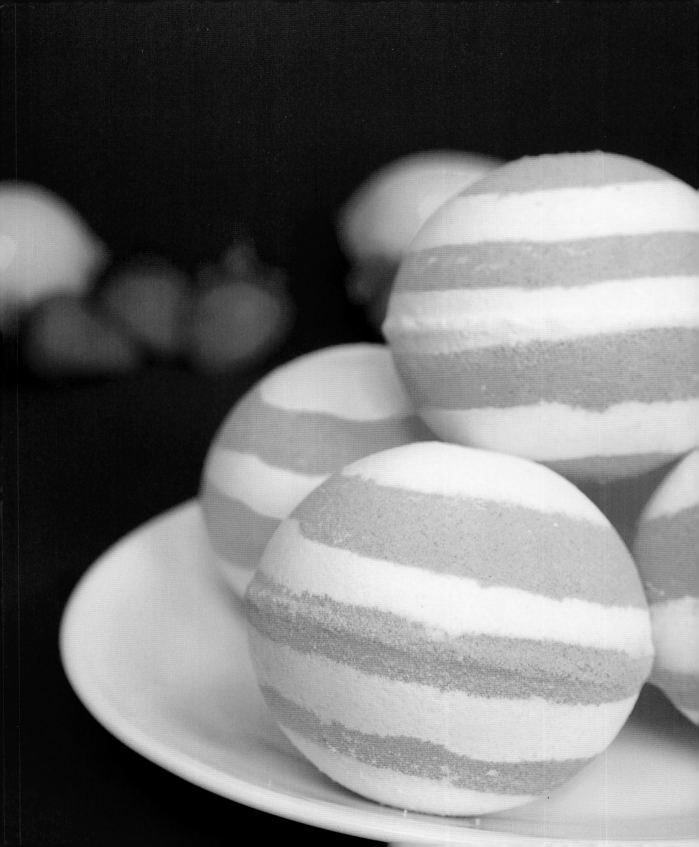

STRAWBERRY LEMONADE
BATH BOMBS

So refreshing in your glass, strawberry lemonade is also a treat when it fizzes your bath. The bright fragrance and colors will delight your senses. Let these bath bombs sweep you away to carefree summer days as your bath water turns a sweet shade of coral!

MAKES

BATH BOMBS

SUPPLIES

3 cups baking soda

1½ tablespoons cream of tartar

2 tablespoons sodium lauryl sulfoacetate (SLSA)

1 teaspoon pink mica colorant

1 teaspoon yellow mica colorant

2 tablespoons sweet almond oil, divided

1 tablespoon polysorbate 80, divided

1 teaspoon strawberry fragrance oil

½ teaspoon lemon essential oil (or 1 teaspoon lemonade fragrance oil)

1½ cups citric acid, divided

Witch hazel, scant amount as needed

2½" round bath bomb mold

MIXING DIRECTIONS

1 · In a large mixing bowl, thoroughly combine the baking soda, cream of tartar, and SLSA. Divide the mixture evenly into two medium bowls. Mix the pink mica into one bowl and the yellow mica into the second bowl.

2 · In a small container, combine 1 tablespoon of the sweet almond oil, ½ tablespoon of the polysorbate 80, and the strawberry fragrance oil. Stirring constantly, slowly mix the liquids into the pink dry ingredients until they are completely combined.

3 · In another small container, combine the remaining sweet almond oil and polysorbate 80 and the lemon essential oil. Stirring constantly, slowly mix the liquids into the yellow dry ingredients until they are completely combined.

4 · Add ¾ cup of the citric acid to each of the bowls and stir until it is fully incorporated into the mixture. If the mixture is not quite wet enough to mold, spritz two to three times with a spray bottle of witch hazel and mix well. Repeat as necessary.

MOLDING DIRECTIONS

5 · Layer the pink and yellow mixtures into both halves of the mold in a striped pattern. Make sure to overfill the mold just a bit. Press the halves firmly together.

6 · Carefully release the bath bomb from the mold and allow it to dry completely for 24–48 hours. Repeat to create the remaining bath bombs.

LEMON POPPYSEED
BATH BOMBS

L *ooking for a classic? Lemon is one of the most well-loved fragrances, known for its uplifting, energizing properties. Fill your tub with the cheery scent and color of citrus fizz that's sure to bring good vibes to your bath time and your entire day!*

MAKES

7

BATH BOMBS

SUPPLIES

1½ cups baking soda

1 tablespoon white kaolin clay

1½ tablespoons sodium lauryl sulfoacetate (SLSA)

½ teaspoon yellow mica colorant

½ teaspoon poppyseeds

1 tablespoon sweet almond oil

1 teaspoon polysorbate 80

25 drops lemon essential oil

¼ teaspoon vanilla fragrance oil

¾ cup citric acid

Witch hazel, scant amount as needed

2″ round bath bomb mold

MIXING DIRECTIONS

1 · In a large mixing bowl, thoroughly combine the baking soda, kaolin clay, SLSA, yellow mica, and poppyseeds.

2 · In a small container, mix together the sweet almond oil, polysorbate 80, lemon essential oil, and vanilla fragrance oil.

3 · Stirring constantly, slowly mix the liquids into the dry ingredients until they are completely combined.

4 · Add the citric acid to the mixture and stir until it is fully incorporated. If the mixture is not quite wet enough to mold, spritz two to three times with a spray bottle of witch hazel and mix well. Repeat as necessary.

MOLDING DIRECTIONS

5 · Lightly overfill both halves of the mold with the mixture. Press the halves firmly together.

6 · Carefully release the bath bomb from the mold and allow it to dry completely for 24–48 hours. Repeat to create the remaining bath bombs.

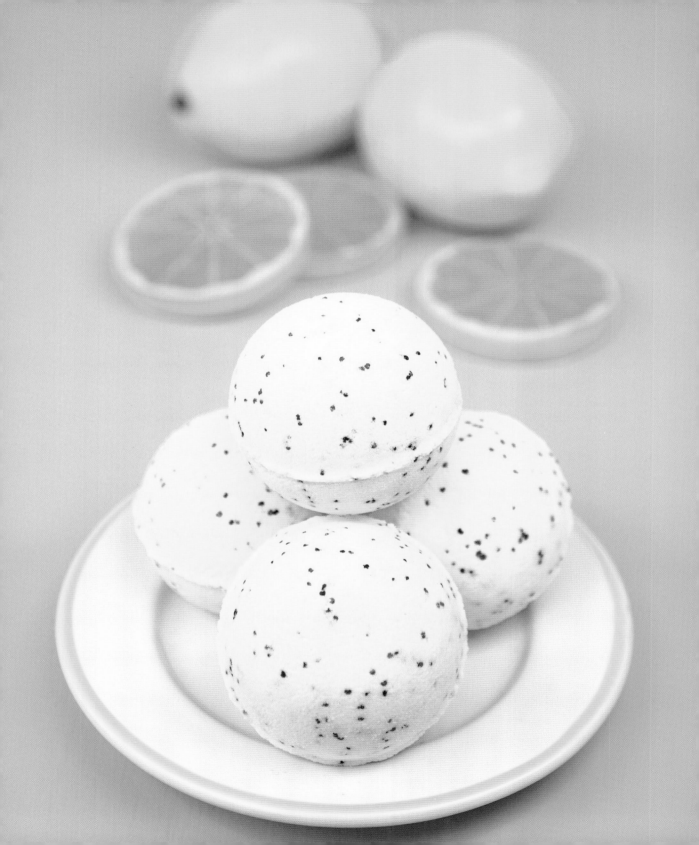

TRIPLE BERRY
BATH BOMBS

*You **can** have it all . . . in your bath! These bath bombs combine three favorite berry fragrances— strawberry, raspberry, and blueberry—into one delightful bath-time treat. Soothe your senses with soft violet-colored fizz and the sweet smell of summertime.*

MAKES

BATH BOMBS

SUPPLIES

3 cups baking soda

1½ tablespoons cream of tartar

2 tablespoons sodium lauryl sulfoacetate (SLSA)

1 teaspoon blue mica colorant

1 teaspoon purple mica colorant

2 tablespoons fractionated coconut oil, divided

1 tablespoon polysorbate 80, divided

½ teaspoon raspberry fragrance oil

½ teaspoon strawberry fragrance oil

½ teaspoon blueberry fragrance oil

1½ cups citric acid, divided

Witch hazel, scant amount as needed

2½″ round bath bomb mold

MIXING DIRECTIONS

1 · In a large mixing bowl, thoroughly combine the baking soda, cream of tartar, and SLSA. Divide the mixture evenly into two medium bowls. Mix the blue mica into one bowl and the purple mica into the second bowl.

2 · In a small container, combine 1 tablespoon of the fractionated coconut oil, ½ tablespoon of the polysorbate 80, raspberry fragrance oil, and strawberry fragrance oil. Stirring constantly, slowly mix the liquids into the purple dry ingredients until they are completely combined.

3 · In another small container, combine the remaining fractionated coconut oil and polysorbate 80 and the blueberry fragrance oil. Stirring constantly, slowly mix the liquids into the blue dry ingredients until they are completely combined.

4 · Add ¾ cup of the citric acid to each of the bowls and stir until it is fully incorporated into the mixture. If the mixture is not quite wet enough to mold, spritz two to three times with a spray bottle of witch hazel and mix well. Repeat as necessary.

MOLDING DIRECTIONS

5 · Fill half of the mold with the blue mixture and the other half with purple. Make sure to overfill the mold just a bit. Press the halves firmly together.

6 · Carefully release the bath bomb from the mold and allow it to dry completely for 24–48 hours. Repeat to create the remaining bath bombs.

GRAPEFRUIT
BATH BOMBS

T reat yourself to a self-care pause with the scent of grapefruit, which has been linked to stress relief, enhanced mood, and positive energy. You'll want to always have a stock of these bath bombs on hand, so you can soak your cares away under soft pink fizz!

MAKES

BATH BOMBS

SUPPLIES

3 cups baking soda

2 tablespoons cream of tartar

2 tablespoons sodium lauryl sulfoacetate (SLSA)

1 teaspoon pink mica colorant

¼ teaspoon yellow mica colorant

2 tablespoons apricot kernel oil

1 tablespoon polysorbate 80

40 drops grapefruit essential oil

1½ cups citric acid

Witch hazel, scant amount as needed

2½" round bath bomb mold

MIXING DIRECTIONS

1 · In a large mixing bowl, thoroughly combine the baking soda, cream of tartar, SLSA, pink mica, and yellow mica.

2 · In a small container, mix together the apricot kernel oil, polysorbate 80, and grapefruit essential oil.

3 · Stirring constantly, slowly mix the liquids into the dry ingredients until they are completely combined.

4 · Add the citric acid to the mixture and stir until it is fully incorporated. If the mixture is not quite wet enough to mold, spritz two to three times with a spray bottle of witch hazel and mix well. Repeat as necessary.

MOLDING DIRECTIONS

5 · Lightly overfill both halves of the mold with the mixture. Press the halves firmly together.

6 · Carefully release the bath bomb from the mold and allow it to dry completely for 24–48 hours. Repeat to create the remaining bath bombs.

STRAWBERRY
BATH BOMBS

With a summery fragrance and sweet effervescence, these strawberries will quickly become a favorite pick! Ease into berry-colored bath water topped with enchanting strawberry suds for a rich and aromatic bath-time experience.

MAKES

BATH BOMBS

SUPPLIES

3 cups baking soda

2 tablespoons cream of tartar

1 tablespoon white kaolin clay

2 tablespoons sodium lauryl sulfoacetate (SLSA)

1 tablespoon red mica colorant

2 tablespoons grapeseed oil

1 tablespoon polysorbate 80

1 teaspoon strawberry fragrance oil

1½ cups citric acid

Witch hazel, scant amount as needed

¼ teaspoon green mica colorant

¼ teaspoon yellow mica colorant

1 teaspoon isopropyl alcohol, divided

Strawberry hard plastic mold

MIXING DIRECTIONS

1 · In a large mixing bowl, thoroughly combine the baking soda, cream of tartar, kaolin clay, SLSA, and red mica.

2 · In a small container, combine the grapeseed oil, polysorbate 80, and strawberry fragrance oil. Stirring constantly, slowly mix the liquids into the dry ingredients until they are completely combined.

3 · Add the citric acid to the mixture and stir until it is fully incorporated. If the mixture is not quite wet enough to mold, spritz two to three times with a spray bottle of witch hazel and mix well. Repeat as necessary.

MOLDING DIRECTIONS

4 · Press the bath bomb mixture firmly into the mold using your thumb and the palm of your hand to apply pressure. Fill the mold to the top until it is packed completely full.

5 · Carefully release the bath bomb from the mold and allow it to dry completely for 24–48 hours. Repeat to create the remaining bath bombs.

6 · When the bath bombs are dry, mix the yellow mica with ½ teaspoon of the isopropyl alcohol and use a small paintbrush to apply the strawberry seed details. Repeat with the green mica and remaining isopropyl alcohol to paint the strawberry stems. Repeat to create the remaining bath bombs.

CHERRY
BATH BOMBS

Toss two of these cherry bombs into your bathtub for a delectable dose of bath-time euphoria! Creamy shea butter and sweet almond oil moisturize your skin as the sweet cherry aroma and abundant soft bubbles nourish your spirit.

MAKES

12

BATH BOMB SETS

SUPPLIES

3 cups baking soda

½ cup Epsom salt, finely ground

2 tablespoons white kaolin clay

2 tablespoons sodium lauryl
    sulfoacetate (SLSA)

1 tablespoon red mica colorant

2 tablespoons sweet almond oil

2 tablespoons shea
    butter, melted

1 tablespoon polysorbate 80

1 teaspoon cherry fragrance oil

1½ cups citric acid

Witch hazel, scant
    amount as needed

1¾" round bath bomb mold

Floral wire, cut into 5" lengths

Green paper

MIXING DIRECTIONS

1 · In a large mixing bowl, thoroughly combine the baking soda, Epsom salt, kaolin clay, SLSA, and red mica.

2 · In a small container, mix together the sweet almond oil, melted shea butter, polysorbate 80, and cherry fragrance oil. Stirring constantly, slowly mix the liquids into the dry ingredients until they are completely combined.

3 · Add the citric acid to the mixture and stir until it is fully incorporated. If the mixture is not quite wet enough to mold, spritz two to three times with a spray bottle of witch hazel and mix well. Repeat as necessary.

MOLDING DIRECTIONS

4 · Lightly overfill both halves of the mold with the mixture. Press the halves firmly together.

5 · Carefully release the bath bomb from the mold. Use the floral wire to poke a small hole in the top. Allow to dry completely for 24–48 hours. Repeat to create the remaining bath bombs.

6 · Bend the floral wire in half and insert each end into a cherry bath bomb. Add a decorative leaf made from green paper.

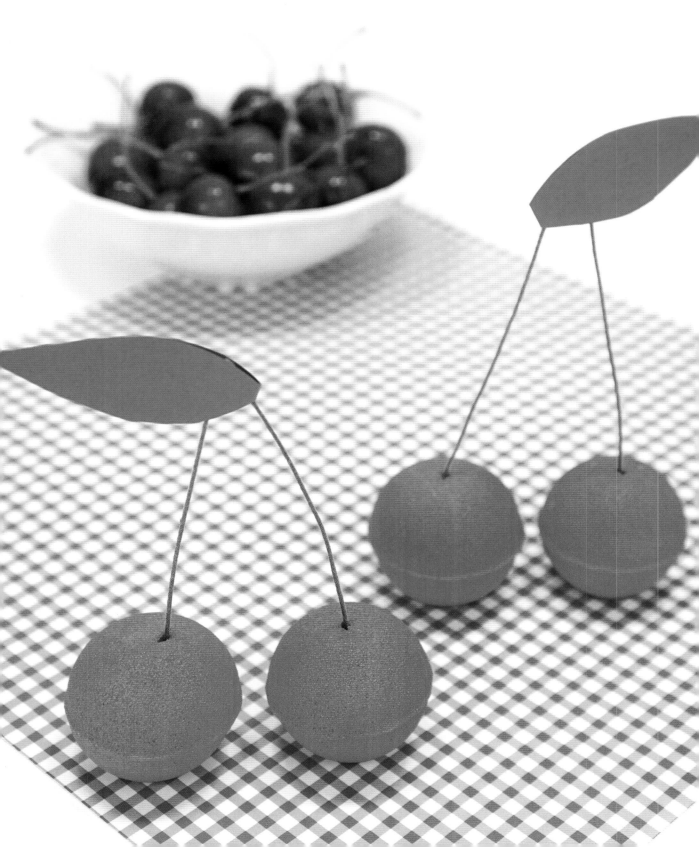

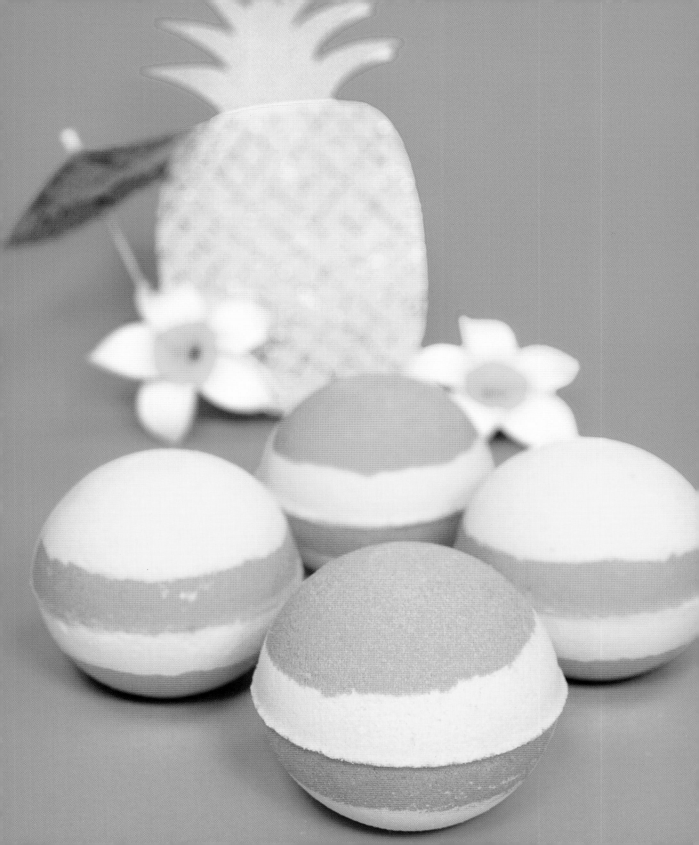

PINEAPPLE-MANGO
BATH BOMBS

Need a sweet escape? These pineapple-mango bath bombs smell like a tropical dream come true! Relax your cares away and drift off to paradise in your own bathtub with piles of fluffy bubbles.

MAKES

BATH BOMBS

SUPPLIES

3 cups baking soda

½ cup Epsom salt, finely ground

2 tablespoons cream of tartar

3 tablespoons sodium lauryl sulfoacetate (SLSA)

½ teaspoon yellow mica colorant

½ teaspoon orange mica colorant

3 tablespoons coconut oil, melted and divided

1 tablespoon polysorbate 80, divided

2 teaspoons cocamidopropyl betaine, divided

1 teaspoon mango fragrance oil

1 teaspoon pineapple fragrance oil

1½ cups citric acid, divided

Witch hazel, scant amount as needed

2½" round bath bomb mold

MIXING DIRECTIONS

1 · In a large mixing bowl, thoroughly combine the baking soda, Epsom salt, cream of tartar, and SLSA. Divide the mixture evenly into two medium bowls. Stir the yellow mica into one bowl and the orange mica into the other.

2 · In a small container, combine 1½ tablespoons of the melted coconut oil, ½ tablespoon of the polysorbate 80, 1 teaspoon of the cocamidopropyl betaine, and the mango fragrance oil. Stirring constantly, slowly mix the liquids into the orange dry ingredients until they are completely combined.

3 · In another small container, combine the remaining coconut oil, polysorbate 80, cocamidopropyl betaine, and pineapple fragrance oil. Stirring constantly, slowly mix the liquids into the yellow dry ingredients until they are completely combined.

4 · Add ¾ cup of the citric acid to each of the bowls and stir until it is fully incorporated into the mixture. If the mixture is not quite wet enough to mold, spritz two to three times with a spray bottle of witch hazel and mix well. Repeat as necessary.

MOLDING DIRECTIONS

5 · Fill both halves of the mold with layers of the yellow and orange mixtures to create stripes. Make sure to overfill the mold just a bit. Press the halves firmly together.

6 · Carefully release the bath bomb from the mold and allow it to dry completely for 24–48 hours. Repeat to create the remaining bath bombs.

GREEN APPLE
BATH BOMBS

Let this crisp scent transport you to the stress-free zone! In fact, the green apple scent has been connected to relief from headaches and anxiety. So settle into a bathtub of calming green and enjoy rejuvenation for your skin and your senses.

MAKES

7

BATH BOMBS

SUPPLIES

1½ cups baking soda

¼ cup cornstarch

2 tablespoons cream of tartar

2 tablespoons sodium lauryl sulfoacetate (SLSA)

½ teaspoon green mica colorant

1 tablespoon fractionated coconut oil

½ tablespoon polysorbate 80

½ tablespoon apple fragrance oil

½ teaspoon water

¾ cups citric acid

Witch hazel, scant amount as needed

2″ round bath bomb mold

Floral wire, cut into 1½″ lengths

Green paper

MIXING DIRECTIONS

1 · In a large mixing bowl, thoroughly combine the baking soda, cornstarch, cream of tartar, SLSA, and green mica.

2 · In a small container, mix together the fractionated coconut oil, polysorbate 80, apple fragrance oil, and water. Stirring constantly, slowly mix the liquids into the dry ingredients until they are completely combined.

3 · Add the citric acid to the mixture and stir until it is fully incorporated. If the mixture is not quite wet enough to mold, spritz two to three times with a spray bottle of witch hazel and mix well. Repeat as necessary.

MOLDING DIRECTIONS

4 · Lightly overfill both halves of the mold with the mixture. Press the halves firmly together.

5 · Carefully release the bath bomb from the mold. Use the floral wire to poke a small hole in the top. Allow to dry completely for 24–48 hours. Repeat to create the remaining bath bombs.

6 · Insert a piece of floral wire into the top of each bath bomb and add a decorative leaf made from green paper.

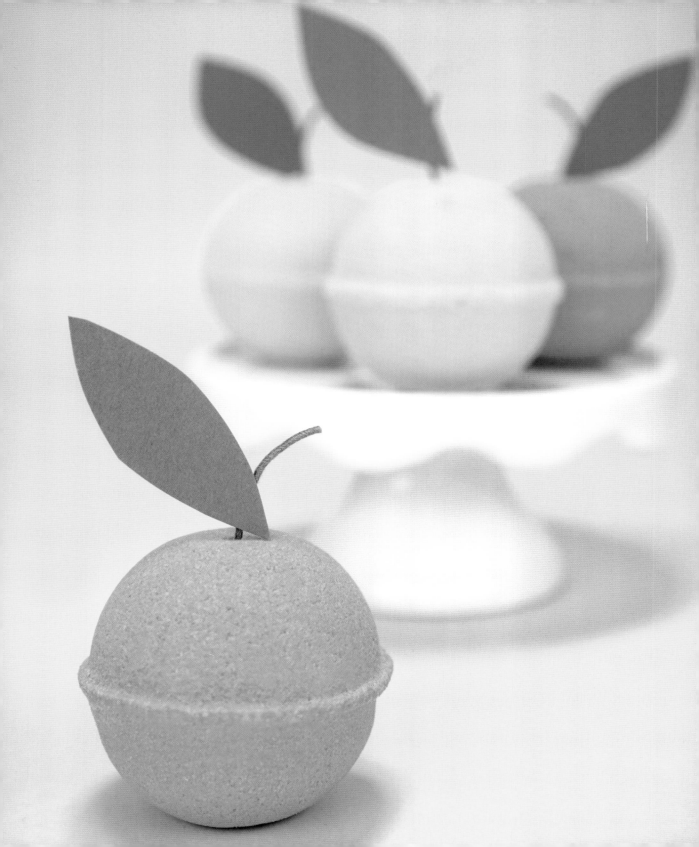

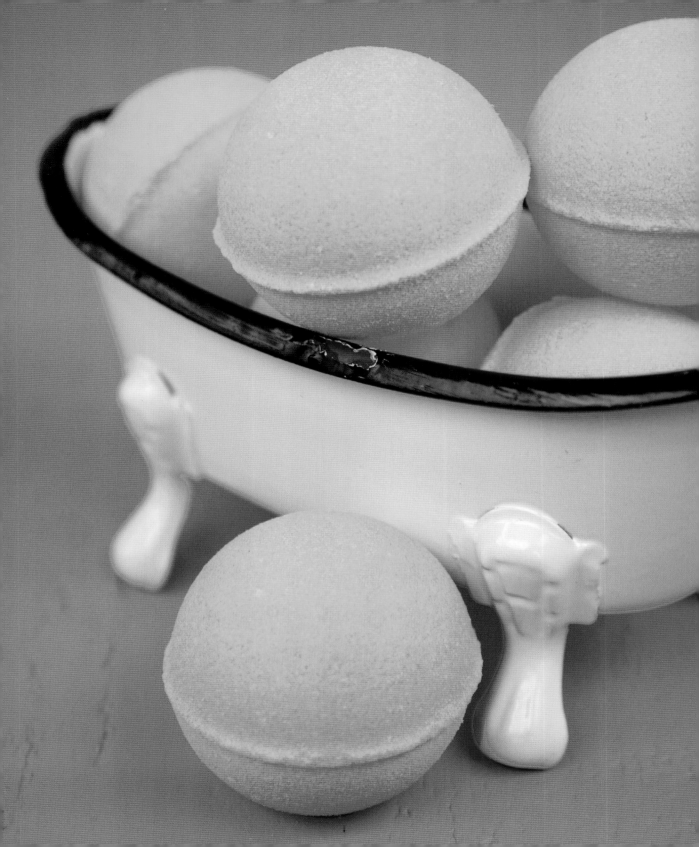

MELON BALL
BATH BOMBS

These pretty little melon balls may look like they belong in a summer fruit salad, but they're a luscious addition to your bath. Indulge in the sweet scent, soft peach-colored water, and a thick, airy layer of moisturizing bubbles.

MAKES

BATH BOMBS

SUPPLIES

1½ cups baking soda

1 tablespoon cream of tartar

1 tablespoon white kaolin clay

⅓ cup cornstarch

1½ tablespoons sodium lauryl sulfoacetate (SLSA)

½ teaspoon coral orange mica colorant

1½ tablespoons fractionated coconut oil

½ tablespoon polysorbate 80

1 teaspoon cocamidopropyl betaine

¼ teaspoon honeydew melon fragrance oil

¼ teaspoon cantaloupe fragrance oil

¾ cup citric acid

Witch hazel, scant amount as needed

2″ round bath bomb mold

MIXING DIRECTIONS

1 · In a large mixing bowl, thoroughly combine the baking soda, cream of tartar, kaolin clay, cornstarch, SLSA, and coral orange mica.

2 · In a small container, mix together the fractionated coconut oil, polysorbate 80, cocamidopropyl betaine, honeydew melon fragrance oil, and cantaloupe fragrance oil.

3 · Stirring constantly, slowly mix the liquids into the dry ingredients until they are completely combined.

4 · Add the citric acid to the mixture and stir until it is fully incorporated. If the mixture is not quite wet enough to mold, spritz two to three times with a spray bottle of witch hazel and mix well. Repeat as necessary.

MOLDING DIRECTIONS

5 · Lightly overfill both halves of the mold with the mixture. Press the halves firmly together.

6 · Carefully release the bath bomb from the mold and allow it to dry completely for 24–48 hours. Repeat to create the remaining bath bombs.

BUBBLING BATH
SCOOPS

Want lots and lots of bubbles? These dreamy scoops will fill your bathtub with mountains of thick, rich, and creamy bubbles. But the benefits go beyond foamy fun. Loaded with moisturizing ingredients, the bath scoops are a treat for your skin.

MAKES

18

BATH SCOOPS

SUPPLIES

2 cups baking soda (plus more as needed)

2 cups sodium lauryl sulfoacetate (SLSA)

⅔ cup cream of tartar

⅔ cup cornstarch

⅔ cup vegetable glycerin

3 tablespoons cocamidopropyl betaine

2 tablespoons sweet almond oil (plus more as needed)

1 teaspoon creamsicle fragrance oil

10 drops pink soap colorant

10 drops yellow soap colorant

10 drops orange soap colorant

2″ ice cream scoop

Small organza mesh bag

MIXING DIRECTIONS

1 · In a large mixing bowl, thoroughly combine the baking soda, SLSA, cream of tartar, and cornstarch.

2 · In a small bowl, mix together the vegetable glycerin, cocamidopropyl betaine, sweet almond oil, and creamsicle fragrance oil. Stirring constantly, slowly mix the liquids into the dry ingredients until they are completely combined to form a soft dough. If the mixture is too sticky, add additional baking soda by the teaspoon until the dough reaches the proper consistency. If the mixture is too dry, add sweet almond oil by the ½ teaspoon.

3 · Divide the dough into three bowls. Add either the pink, yellow, or orange soap colorant to each. Knead the dough until the color is completely incorporated.

4 · Place all three pieces of dough side by side to form one larger piece of dough. Use the ice cream scoop to scoop across all three colors of dough as you form your bubble bath scoop.

5 · Place the bubble bath scoops on a sheet of parchment paper or a silicone mat and allow to dry completely. Drying can take from 3–7 days depending on temperature and humidity.

To use · Crumble the scoop into small pieces and place it inside the mesh bag. Hold the bag under running bath water to create luxurious bubbles in your tub! Use half of the bubble scoop for a tub full of bubbles or a full scoop for a truly outrageous bath-time experience.

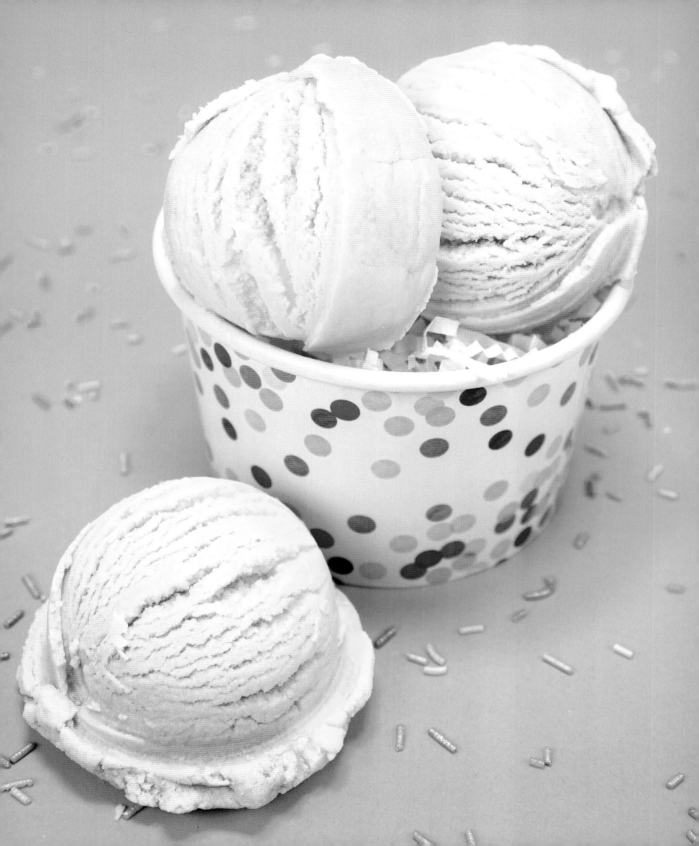

WATERMELON
SOAPS

Deliciously scented and delightfully whimsical, this watermelon soap is much more than eye candy. It will keep your skin refreshed, moisturized, and exfoliated with a combination of goat's milk, glycerin, and a sprinkle of poppyseeds.

MAKES

12

SOAPS

SUPPLIES

1 pound goat's milk soap base, sliced into cubes

Microwave-safe measuring cup(s)

60 drops watermelon fragrance oil, divided

10 drops green soap colorant

42-ounce silicone loaf soap mold

Isopropyl alcohol, in a spray bottle

2 pounds crystal clear glycerin suspension soap base, sliced into cubes

15 drops red soap colorant

1 teaspoon poppyseeds

DIRECTIONS

1 · To make the dark green layer: Place ½ pound of the goat's milk soap base cubes into a microwave-safe measuring cup. Melt the soap in the microwave in 30-second increments, stirring well after each session to ensure that it is completely melted. Add 10 drops of the watermelon fragrance oil and the green soap colorant and mix well.

2 · Pour ¾ of the melted soap into the bottom of the soap mold and spritz the top with isopropyl alcohol to remove any air bubbles. Allow to firm for 15 minutes.

3 · To make the light green layer: Take the remaining dark green soap (still in the measuring cup) and add ¼ pound of the goat's milk soap base cubes. Melt in the microwave in 30-second increments, stirring well after each session to ensure that the soap is completely melted. Add 10 drops of the watermelon fragrance oil.

4 · Spritz the top of the dark green soap layer with isopropyl alcohol (to help the layers stick together), pour the melted light green soap into the mold, and spritz the top with isopropyl alcohol to remove any air bubbles. Allow to firm for 15 minutes.

5 · To make the white layer: Place the remaining ¼ pound goat's milk soap base into a clean microwave-safe measuring cup. Melt in the microwave in 30-second increments, stirring well after each session to ensure that the soap is completely melted. Add 10 drops of the watermelon fragrance oil.

$6\cdot$ Spritz the top of the light green layer with isopropyl alcohol, pour the white soap into the mold, and spritz the top with isopropyl alcohol to remove any air bubbles. Allow to firm for 15 minutes.

$7\cdot$ *To make the red layer:* Place the crystal clear glycerin suspension soap base into a clean microwave-safe measuring cup. Melt in the microwave in 30-second increments, stirring well after each session to ensure that the soap is completely melted. Add 30 drops of the watermelon fragrance oil, the red soap colorant, and poppyseeds, and mix well.

$8\cdot$ Spritz the top of the white layer with isopropyl alcohol, pour the red soap into the mold, and spritz the top with isopropyl alcohol to remove any air bubbles. Allow to sit undisturbed until completely cooled and firm (2–24 hours depending on temperature and humidity).

$9\cdot$ Once the loaf of soap is cooled, carefully remove it from the silicone mold. Use a sharp knife to slice the loaf into individual soaps.

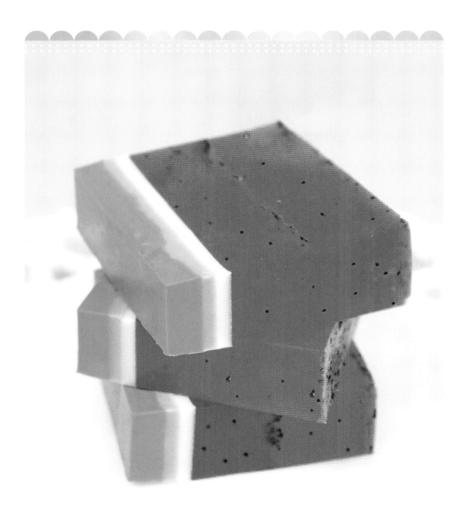

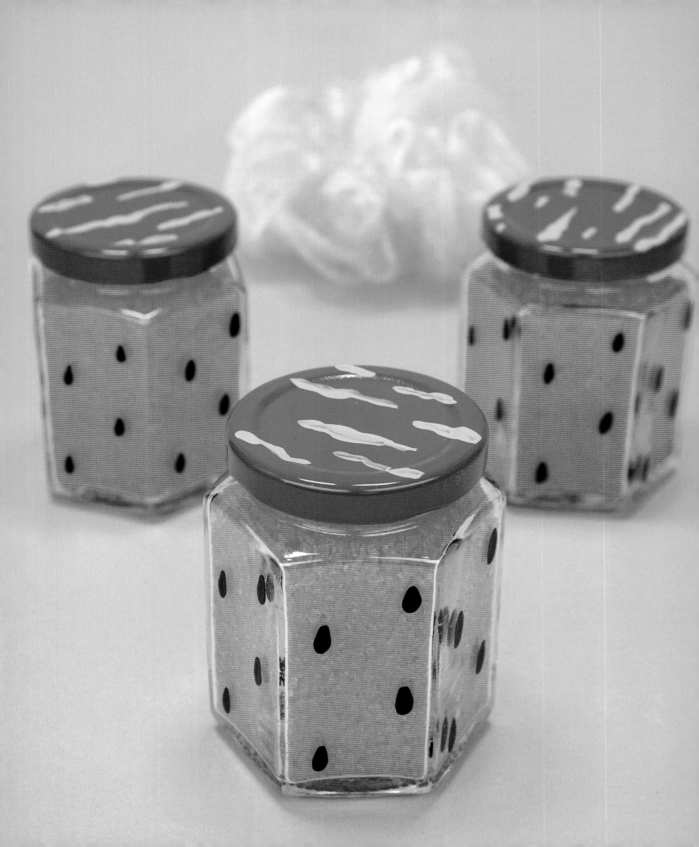

WATERMELON
BATH SALTS

Soak away your worries and your sore muscles with an easy, four-ingredient recipe! Epsom salt is known to soothe muscle aches, relieve tension, and detoxify the skin. Add these bath salts to your tub for a relaxing and healing treatment for the mind and body.

MAKES

8 OUNCES

BATH SALTS

SUPPLIES

1 cup Epsom salt

½ teaspoon polysorbate 80

¼ teaspoon watermelon
  fragrance oil

⅛ teaspoon bright pink
  mica colorant

Glass storage container with lid

Acrylic paint in dark green,
  light green, and black

DIRECTIONS

1 · In a small bowl, mix together the Epsom salt, polysorbate 80, watermelon fragrance oil, and pink mica. Allow the colored salts to dry for at least an hour.

2 · Place the salts in a glass storage container and seal. Use the paint to add watermelon details to the jar.

To use · Empty the contents of the jar into warm running bath water. Soak for at least 20 minutes for best results.

SHIMMERY GRAPEFRUIT
SOAPS

*G*rapefruit has long been used as a skin-brightening and antiaging treatment, and these shimmery grapefruit soaps pack all the benefits into one pretty package! Exfoliate, detox, smooth, and brighten with this antioxidant-rich skin treatment.

MAKES

SOAPS

SUPPLIES

Pearl mica cosmetic
  shimmer powder

Decorative round
  silicone soap mold

1 pound shea butter soap base

Microwave-safe measuring cup

5 drops orange soap colorant

2 drops pink soap colorant

30 drops grapefruit essential oil

Isopropyl alcohol, in
  a spray bottle

DIRECTIONS

1 · Use a paintbrush to apply a thin layer of pearl mica shimmer powder to the bottom of the soap molds.

2 · Slice the shea butter soap base into small cubes and place into a microwave-safe measuring cup. Melt in the microwave in 30-second increments, stirring well after each session to ensure that the soap is completely melted.

3 · Carefully stir in the orange soap colorant, pink soap colorant, and grapefruit essential oil.

4 · Pour the melted soap into the mold and spritz with isopropyl alcohol to remove any air bubbles.

5 · Allow the soaps to sit undisturbed until completely firm (approximately 60–90 minutes depending on temperature and humidity) before unmolding.

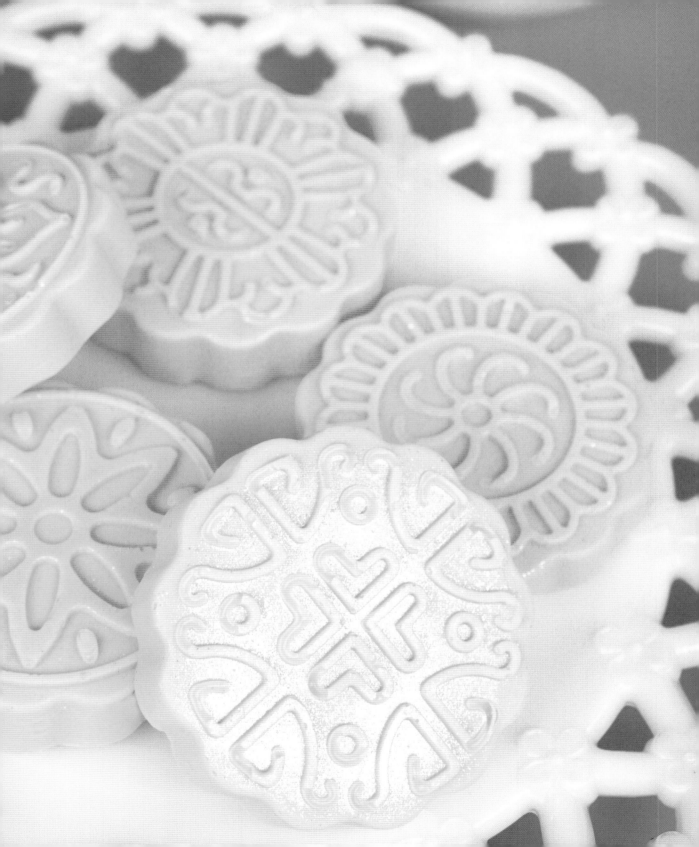

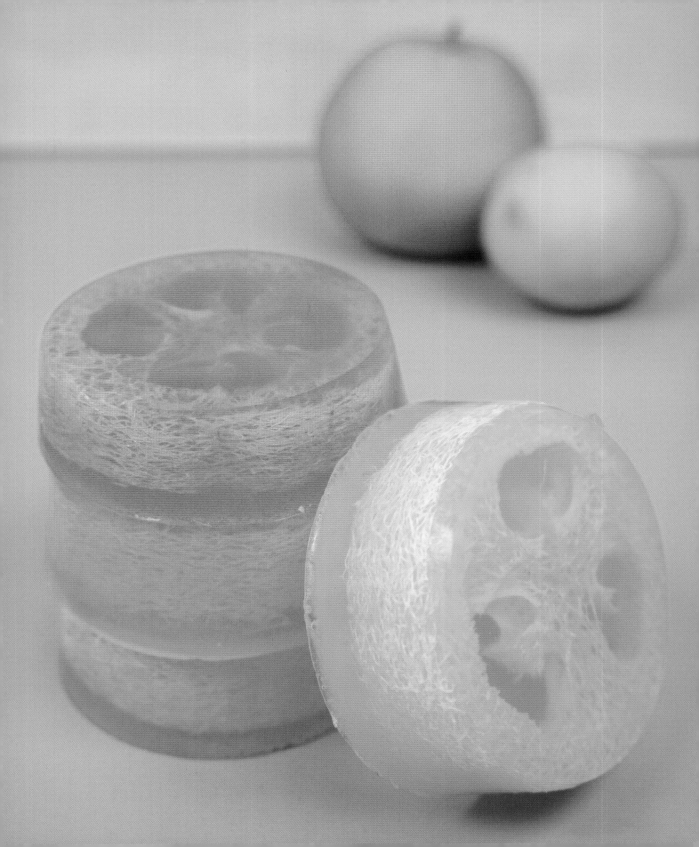

CITRUS LOOFAH
SOAPS

These refreshing soaps are a fantastic way to exfoliate and rehydrate dry skin! Keep your skin feeling smooth and silky all year long with natural loofah and a blend of citrus oils. As a bonus, the cheerful colors brighten up any place you display them.

MAKES

SOAPS

SUPPLIES

Serrated knife

Natural loofah

Round silicone soap mold

1 pound crystal clear glycerin soap base, cubed

Microwave-safe measuring cup

6 drops yellow soap colorant

30 drops citrus blend essential oil

Isopropyl alcohol, in a spray bottle

9 drops orange soap colorant, divided

DIRECTIONS

1 · With the serrated knife, cut 1" thick slices of the loofah. Place a slice into the bottom of each well in the mold.

2 · Place the soap base cubes into a microwave-safe measuring cup. Melt in the microwave in 30-second increments, stirring well after each session to ensure that the soap is completely melted.

3 · Carefully stir the yellow soap colorant and citrus essential oil into the melted soap.

4 · Pour the mixture into two wells of the mold. Spritz with isopropyl alcohol to remove any air bubbles.

5 · Reheat the remaining soap if necessary and add 3 drops of the orange soap colorant. Pour into two wells of the mold and spritz with isopropyl alcohol.

6 · Add the remaining orange colorant to the remaining melted soap. Pour into the last two wells of the mold. Spritz with isopropyl alcohol.

7 · Allow the soaps to sit undisturbed until completely firm (approximately 60–90 minutes depending on temperature and humidity) before unmolding.

PIÑA COLADA
SUGAR SCRUB

Say goodbye to dull, dry skin with this pretty and powerful DIY exfoliator! The bright fragrance of this gentle sugar scrub will delight your senses while leaving your skin feeling clean, smooth, and ready to take on the world.

MAKES

10 OUNCES

SUGAR SCRUB

SUPPLIES

1 cup granulated sugar

⅛ teaspoon gold or
   yellow mica colorant

½ cup coconut oil, melted

15 drops pineapple
   fragrance oil

Storage jars

DIRECTIONS

1 · Pour the sugar into a medium-sized bowl. Add the mica to the sugar and stir until well combined.

2 · In a small bowl, melt the coconut oil. Add the pineapple fragrance oil.

3 · Mix the liquid ingredients into the dry ingredients until thoroughly combined.

4 · Store in an air-tight jar or container.

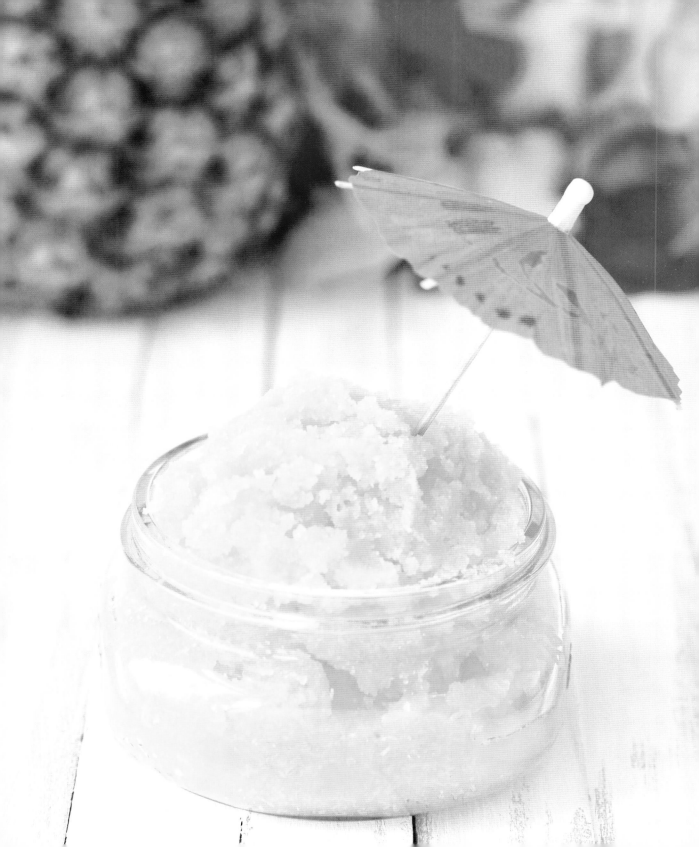

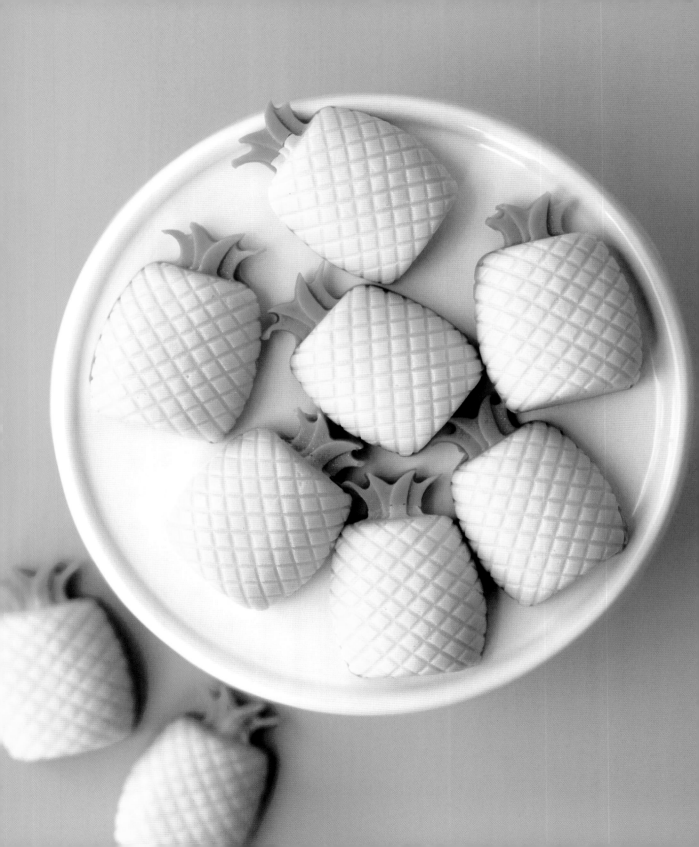

PINEAPPLE
MINI SOAPS

Do you like piña coladas? You'll love these sweet-scented pineapple soaps! Whisk yourself away to a tropical paradise every time you lather up with these luxurious coconut milk–based soaps.

SUPPLIES

½ pound coconut milk soap base

Microwave-safe measuring cup

6 drops gold soap colorant

20 drops pineapple fragrance oil

2 silicone pineapple ice cube trays

Isopropyl alcohol, in a spray bottle

10 drops green soap colorant

DIRECTIONS

1 · Slice the coconut milk soap base into small cubes and place into a microwave-safe measuring cup. Melt in the microwave in 30-second increments, stirring well after each session to ensure that the soap is completely melted.

2 · Carefully stir in the gold soap colorant and pineapple fragrance oil. Pour the melted soap into the wells of the mold, filling each about ⅔ of the way full (up to the leaves), and spritz with isopropyl alcohol to remove any air bubbles. (Note: there will still be gold soap remaining in the measuring cup.) Allow to cool for 15 minutes.

3 · Remelt the remaining gold soap in the measuring cup and add the green soap colorant. Pour the melted green soap into the leaf area of the molds (fill to the top) and spritz with isopropyl alcohol to remove any bubbles.

4 · Allow the soaps to sit undisturbed until completely firm (approximately 20–60 minutes depending on temperature and humidity) before unmolding.

MACARON
SOAPS

Made with a rich and luxurious goat's milk soap base, these sweet soaps leave your skin feeling fresh and silky smooth. Get creative by customizing the soaps with your favorite color and fragrance combinations—or combos that suit a gift recipient!

MAKES

SOAPS

SUPPLIES

1 pound goat's milk soap base

2 microwave-safe measuring cups

10 drops pink soap colorant

15 drops raspberry fragrance oil

Silicone macaron soap mold

Isopropyl alcohol, in a spray bottle

15 drops French vanilla fragrance oil

DIRECTIONS

1 · Slice the goat milk's soap base into small cubes and set aside ⅛ pound of cubes. Place the remaining cubes into a microwave-safe measuring cup. Melt in the microwave in 30-second increments, stirring well after each session to ensure that the soap is completely melted.

2 · Carefully stir in the pink soap colorant and raspberry fragrance oil. Pour the melted soap into the wells of the mold, filling each about ⅓ of the way full (up to the filling line), and spritz with isopropyl alcohol to remove any air bubbles. (Note: there will still be pink soap remaining in the measuring cup.) Allow to cool for 20 minutes.

4 · In another small microwave-safe measuring cup, melt the remaining ⅛ pound of soap cubes. Carefully stir the French vanilla fragrance oil into the melted soap. Spritz the top of the pink soap layer with isopropyl alcohol (to help the layers stick together), pour the white layer of soap "filling" into the molds, and spritz with isopropyl alcohol to remove any bubbles. Allow to cool for 15 minutes.

5 · Remelt the remaining pink soap in the measuring cup. Spritz the top of the white layer of soap with isopropyl alcohol, pour the remaining pink soap into the molds, and spritz with isopropyl alcohol to remove any bubbles.

6 · Allow the soaps to sit undisturbed until completely firm (approximately 30–90 minutes depending on temperature and humidity) before unmolding.

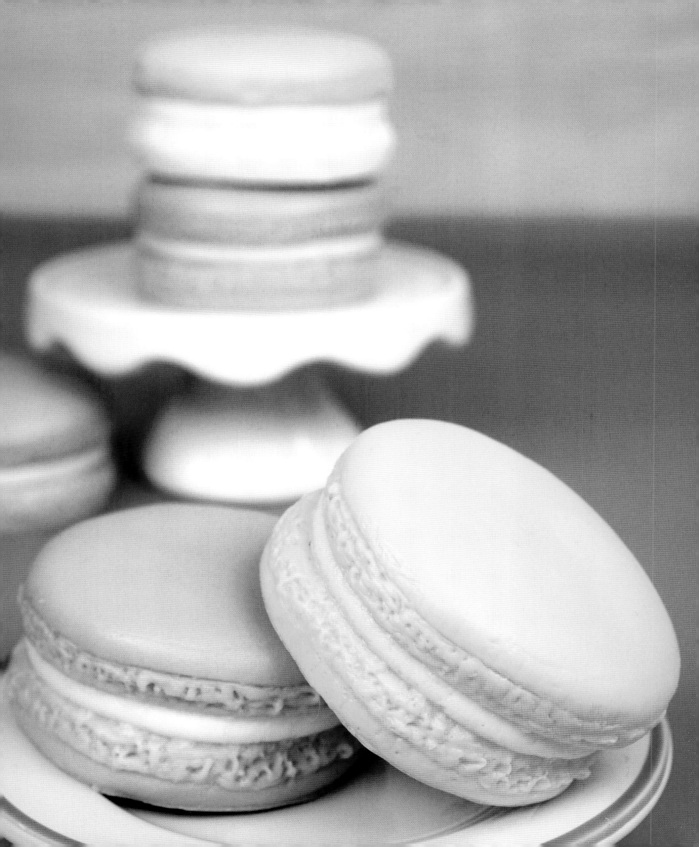

SUGAR COOKIE
BODY BUTTER

Treat yourself to this creamy body butter and infuse your skin with the healing benefits of coconut oil, shea butter, and sweet almond oil, which include antiaging, cellulite-smoothing, and acne-fighting properties. Plus, it smells **amazing!**

MAKES

10 OUNCES

BODY BUTTER

SUPPLIES

⅓ cup coconut oil

⅓ cup shea butter

2 tablespoons sweet almond oil

30 drops sugar cookie fragrance oil

Stainless steel or other heatproof mixing bowl

Mixer

Storage jars

DIRECTIONS

1 · Place a mixing bowl in the refrigerator to chill for at least 30 minutes.

2 · In a small saucepan, melt the coconut oil and shea butter over low heat. When melted, remove from the heat and add the sweet almond oil and sugar cookie fragrance oil.

3 · Carefully pour the liquid into a chilled bowl and allow to sit until the oils begin to harden. You can speed up the process by placing the bowl back into the refrigerator, but be careful not to let it get too hard! You want the oils to be firm, but not solid, for the next step (about the consistency of softened butter).

4 · When the mixture is ready, whip with a mixer for several minutes until the body butter becomes fluffy and the volume has increased. Store in an airtight jar or container.

NATURE'S

BEAUTY

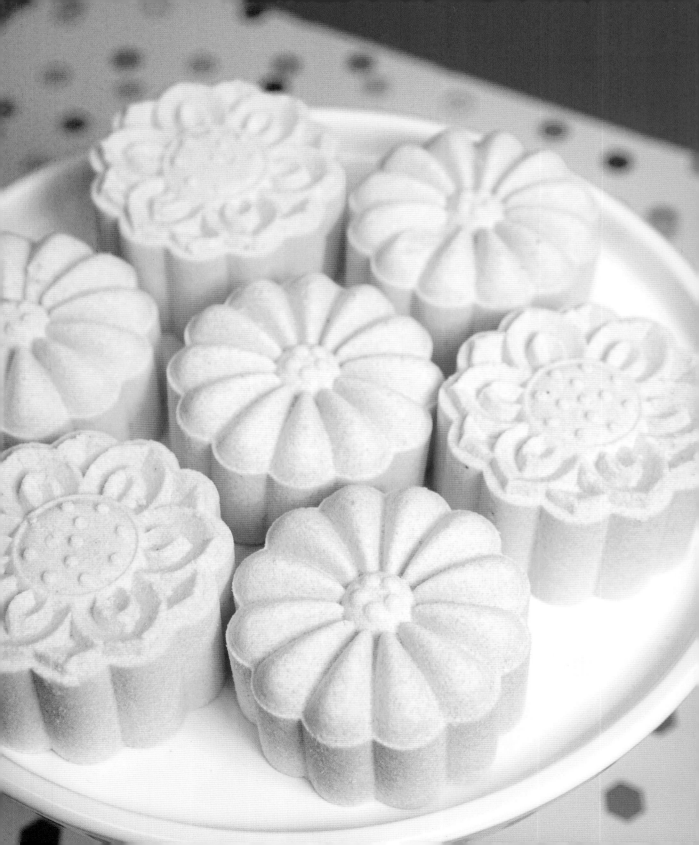

MOONCAKE
BATH BOMBS

These gorgeous, jasmine-scented bath bombs use a traditional Chinese mooncake mold to create delicate and intricate flowers. The pleasing fragrance and color will calm your stress. In fact, jasmine has been used for hundreds of years as a natural means for improving mood and balancing hormones.

MAKES

14

BATH BOMBS

SUPPLIES

3 cups baking soda

1½ tablespoons white kaolin clay

1½ tablespoons sodium lauryl sulfoacetate (SLSA)

1 teaspoon pink mica colorant

2 tablespoons sweet almond oil

1 tablespoon polysorbate 80

15 drops jasmine essential oil or fragrance oil

1½ cups citric acid

Witch hazel, scant amount as needed

Cyclomethicone liquid, for coating mold

65g cookie-press mooncake mold

MIXING DIRECTIONS

1 · In a large mixing bowl, thoroughly combine the baking soda, kaolin clay, SLSA, and pink mica.

2 · In a small container, stir together the sweet almond oil, polysorbate 80, and jasmine oil. Stirring constantly, slowly add the liquids into the dry ingredients until they are completely combined.

3 · Add the citric acid to the mixture and stir until it is fully incorporated. If the mixture is not quite wet enough to mold, spritz two to three times with a spray bottle of witch hazel and mix well. Repeat as necessary.

MOLDING DIRECTIONS

4 · To allow for easy release, brush the inside of the mold with cyclomethicone liquid.

5 · Press the bath bomb mixture firmly into the mold using your thumb and the palm of your hand to apply pressure. Fill the mold to the top until it is packed full. Use the plunger to gently expel the bath bomb from the mold. Repeat with the remaining mixture, re-treating with cyclomethicone liquid as needed.

6 · Allow each bomb to dry completely for 24–48 hours.

SUNFLOWER
BATH BOMBS

Sunflowers are more than just pretty! Sunflower oil is loaded with antioxidant vitamin E and boasts skin benefits ranging from calming irritation to healing acne. As you soak in bright, sunny yellow bath water, you'll soothe your skin under a layer of fizzy bubbles.

MAKES

8

BATH BOMBS

SUPPLIES

1½ cups baking soda

2 tablespoons cream of tartar

1½ tablespoons sodium
  lauryl sulfoacetate (SLSA)

½ teaspoon yellow
  mica colorant

2 tablespoons sunflower oil

½ tablespoon polysorbate 80

½ teaspoon sunflower
  fragrance oil

¾ cup citric acid

Witch hazel, scant
  amount as needed

Hard plastic sunflower
  bath bomb mold

⅛ teaspoon copper
  brown mica colorant

¼ teaspoon isopropyl alcohol

MIXING DIRECTIONS

1· In a large mixing bowl, thoroughly combine the baking soda, cream of tartar, SLSA, and yellow mica.

2· In a small container, mix together the sunflower oil, polysorbate 80, and sunflower fragrance oil. Stirring constantly, slowly mix the liquids into the dry ingredients until they are completely combined.

3· Add the citric acid to the mixture and stir until it is fully incorporated. If the mixture is not quite wet enough to mold, spritz two to three times with a spray bottle of witch hazel and mix well. Repeat as necessary.

MOLDING DIRECTIONS

4· Press the bath bomb mixture firmly into the mold using your thumb and the palm of your hand to apply pressure. Fill the mold to the top until it is packed completely full.

5· Carefully release the bath bomb from the mold and allow it to dry completely for 24–48 hours. Repeat to create the remaining bath bombs.

6· When the bath bombs are dry, mix the copper brown mica with the isopropyl alcohol. Use a small paintbrush to apply detail to the center of the flowers.

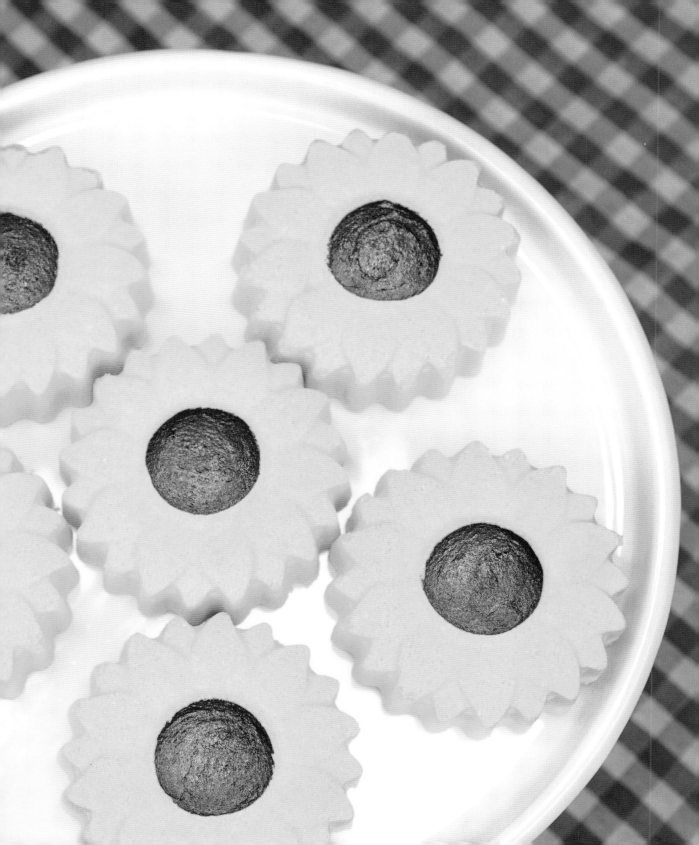

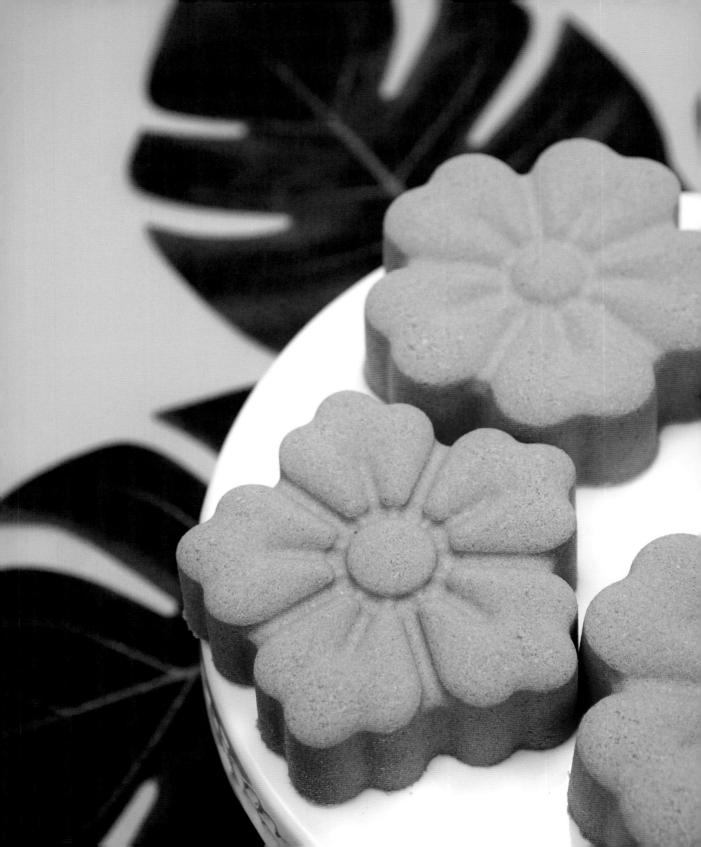

HIBISCUS
BATH BOMBS

Sometimes called "the Botox plant," hibiscus is a treasured natural beauty resource known for treating acne, dark circles, skin discoloration, and aging. These hibiscus bath bombs will infuse your bath with sweetly scented lavender water and leave your skin feeling vibrant and refreshed.

MAKES

BATH BOMBS

SUPPLIES

3 cups baking soda

½ cup cornstarch

½ cup Epsom salt, finely ground

2 tablespoons cream of tartar

2 tablespoons white kaolin clay

2 tablespoons sodium lauryl sulfoacetate (SLSA)

1 teaspoon purple mica colorant

2 tablespoons sweet almond oil

2 tablespoons shea butter, melted

1 tablespoon polysorbate 80

25 drops hibiscus essential oil

1½ cups citric acid

Witch hazel, scant amount as needed

Hard plastic hibiscus bath bomb mold

MIXING DIRECTIONS

1 · In a large mixing bowl, thoroughly combine the baking soda, cornstarch, Epsom salt, cream of tartar, kaolin clay, SLSA, and purple mica.

2 · In a small container, mix together the sweet almond oil, melted shea butter, polysorbate 80, and hibiscus essential oil. Stirring constantly, slowly mix the liquids into the dry ingredients until they are completely combined.

3 · Add the citric acid to the mixture and stir until it is fully incorporated. If the mixture is not quite wet enough to mold, spritz two to three times with a spray bottle of witch hazel and mix well. Repeat as necessary.

MOLDING DIRECTIONS

4 · Press the bath bomb mixture firmly into the mold using your thumb and the palm of your hand to apply pressure. Fill the mold to the top until it is packed completely full.

5 · Carefully release the bath bomb from the mold and allow it to dry completely for 24–48 hours. Repeat to create the remaining bath bombs.

CHERRY BLOSSOM
BATH BOMBS

In Japanese culture, cherry blossoms symbolize the birth of springtime as well as the extreme beauty and fragility of life. The ephemeral beauty of these delicate cherry blossom bath bombs will fill your bathtub with dreamy pink water and a light layer of foam to hydrate your skin.

MAKES

BATH BOMBS

SUPPLIES

1½ cups baking soda

2 tablespoons white kaolin clay

2 tablespoons milk powder

½ teaspoon coral pink
  mica colorant

1 tablespoon fractionated
  coconut oil

1 tablespoon shea
  butter, melted

½ tablespoon polysorbate 80

½ teaspoon Japanese cherry
  blossom fragrance oil

¾ cup citric acid

Witch hazel, scant
  amount as needed

Cyclomethicone liquid,
  for coating mold

50g cherry blossom
  mooncake mold

MIXING DIRECTIONS

1 · In a large mixing bowl, thoroughly combine the baking soda, kaolin clay, milk powder, and coral pink mica.

2 · In a small container, mix together the fractionated coconut oil, melted shea butter, polysorbate 80, and Japanese cherry blossom fragrance oil. Stirring constantly, slowly mix the liquids into the dry ingredients until they are completely combined.

3 · Add the citric acid to the mixture and stir until it is fully incorporated. If the mixture is not quite wet enough to mold, spritz two to three times with a spray bottle of witch hazel and mix well. Repeat as necessary.

MOLDING DIRECTIONS

4 · To allow for easy release, brush the inside of the mold with cyclomethicone liquid.

5 · Press the bath bomb mixture firmly into the mold using your thumb and the palm of your hand to apply pressure. Fill the mold to the top until it is packed full. Use the plunger to gently expel the bath bomb from the mold. Repeat with the remaining mixture, re-treating with cyclomethicone liquid as needed.

6 · Allow each bomb to dry completely for 24–48 hours.

DAFFODIL
BATH BOMBS

Daffodils are symbols of new beginnings and hope, so let these daffodil bath bombs steal away your stress and fill your heart with dreams. Grapeseed oil will bathe your skin in luxurious moisture, while lily essential oil helps reduce anxiety and tension.

MAKES

4

BATH BOMBS

SUPPLIES

1½ cups baking soda

½ cup cornstarch

2 tablespoons arrowroot powder

1 tablespoon sodium lauryl sulfoacetate (SLSA)

½ teaspoon yellow mica colorant

1 tablespoon grapeseed oil

½ tablespoon polysorbate 80

½ teaspoon vegetable glycerin

½ teaspoon lily essential oil

¾ cup citric acid

Witch hazel, scant amount as needed

Hard plastic daffodil bath bomb mold

MIXING DIRECTIONS

1 · In a large mixing bowl, thoroughly combine the baking soda, cornstarch, arrowroot powder, SLSA, and yellow mica.

2 · In a small container, mix together grapeseed oil, polysorbate 80, vegetable glycerin, and lily essential oil. Stirring constantly, slowly mix the liquids into the dry ingredients until they are completely combined.

3 · Add the citric acid to the mixture and stir until it is fully incorporated. If the mixture is not quite wet enough to mold, spritz two to three times with a spray bottle of witch hazel and mix well. Repeat as necessary.

MOLDING DIRECTIONS

4 · Press the bath bomb mixture firmly into the mold using your thumb and the palm of your hand to apply pressure. Fill the mold to the top until it is packed completely full.

5 · Carefully release the bath bomb from the mold and allow it to dry completely for 24–48 hours. Repeat to create the remaining bath bombs.

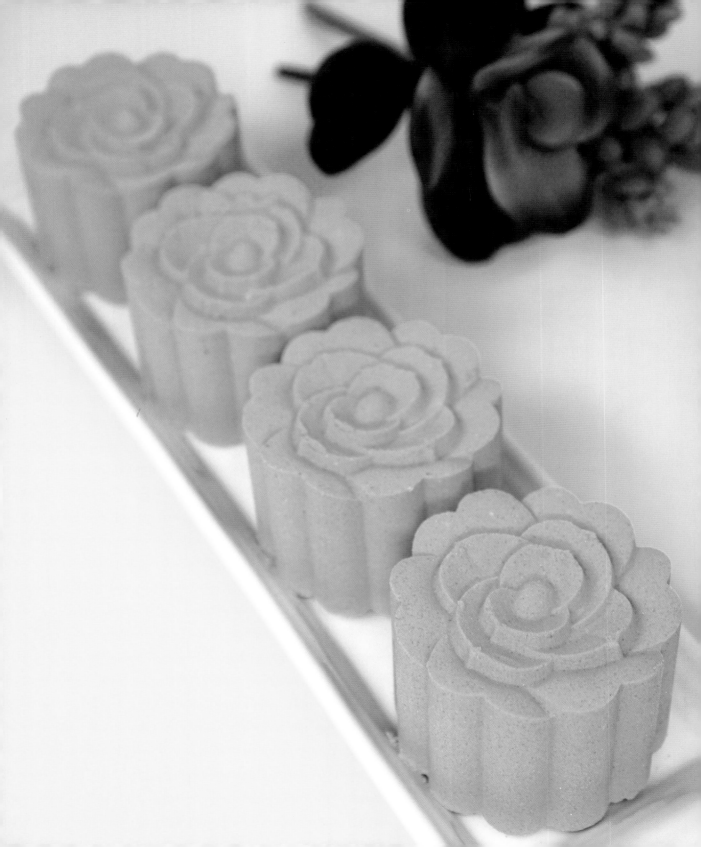

SUCCULENT
BATH BOMBS

*L*oaded with B-complex vitamins and vitamin E,
jojoba oil is one of the best natural moisturizers
for skin and can help soothe skin ailments like eczema
and rosacea. These bath bombs will also calm your
mind with spa-like scents and aqua-colored bubbles.

MAKES

14

BATH BOMBS

SUPPLIES

3 cups baking soda

1½ tablespoons bentonite clay

1½ tablespoons
arrowroot powder

1½ tablespoons sodium
lauryl sulfoacetate (SLSA)

1 teaspoon teal mica colorant

2 tablespoons jojoba oil

1 tablespoon polysorbate 80

1 teaspoon cucumber
melon fragrance oil

1½ cups citric acid

Witch hazel, scant
amount as needed

Cyclomethicone liquid,
for coating mold

65g cookie-press succulent
mooncake mold

MIXING DIRECTIONS

1 · In a large mixing bowl, thoroughly combine the baking soda, bentonite clay, arrowroot powder, SLSA, and teal mica.

2 · In a small container, stir together the jojoba oil, polysorbate 80, and cucumber melon fragrance oil. Stirring constantly, slowly add the liquids into the dry ingredients until they are completely combined.

3 · Add the citric acid to the mixture and stir until it is fully incorporated. If the mixture is not quite wet enough to mold, spritz two to three times with a spray bottle of witch hazel and mix well. Repeat as necessary.

MOLDING DIRECTIONS

4 · To allow for easy release, brush the inside of the mold with cyclomethicone liquid.

5 · Press the bath bomb mixture firmly into the mold using your thumb and the palm of your hand to apply pressure. Fill the mold to the top until it is packed full. Use the plunger to gently expel the bath bomb from the mold. Repeat with the remaining mixture, re-treating with cyclomethicone liquid as needed.

6 · Allow each bomb to dry completely for 24–48 hours.

TURTLE
BATH BOMBS

These adorable turtles are packed with skin-boosting benefits, thanks to the addition of rich avocado oil and vegetable glycerin. Avocado has long been used as an at-home beauty treatment, and this winning combination of ingredients will help skin feel soft and look youthful.

MAKES

BATH BOMBS

SUPPLIES

3 cups baking soda

2 tablespoons cream of tartar

2 tablespoons white kaolin clay

2½ tablespoons sodium lauryl sulfoacetate (SLSA)

1 teaspoon green mica colorant

2 tablespoons avocado oil

1 tablespoon polysorbate 80

1 teaspoon ocean breeze fragrance oil

½ teaspoon vegetable glycerin

1½ cups citric acid

Witch hazel, scant amount as needed

Hard plastic turtle bath bomb mold

MIXING DIRECTIONS

1 · In a large mixing bowl, thoroughly combine the baking soda, cream of tartar, kaolin clay, SLSA, and green mica.

2 · In a small container, stir together the avocado oil, polysorbate 80, ocean breeze fragrance oil, and vegetable glycerin. Stirring constantly, slowly add the liquids into the dry ingredients until they are completely combined.

3 · Add the citric acid to the mixture and stir until it is fully incorporated. If the mixture is not quite wet enough to mold, spritz two to three times with a spray bottle of witch hazel and mix well. Repeat as necessary.

MOLDING DIRECTIONS

4 · Press the bath bomb mixture firmly into the mold using your thumb and the palm of your hand to apply pressure. Fill the mold to the top until it is packed completely full.

5 · Carefully release the bath bomb from the mold and allow it to dry completely for 24–48 hours. Repeat to create the remaining bath bombs.

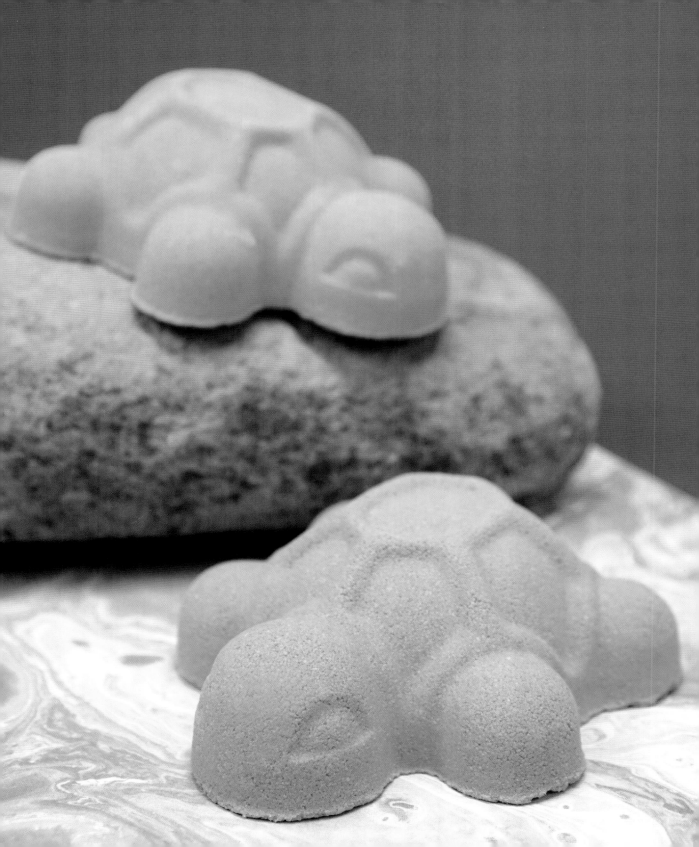

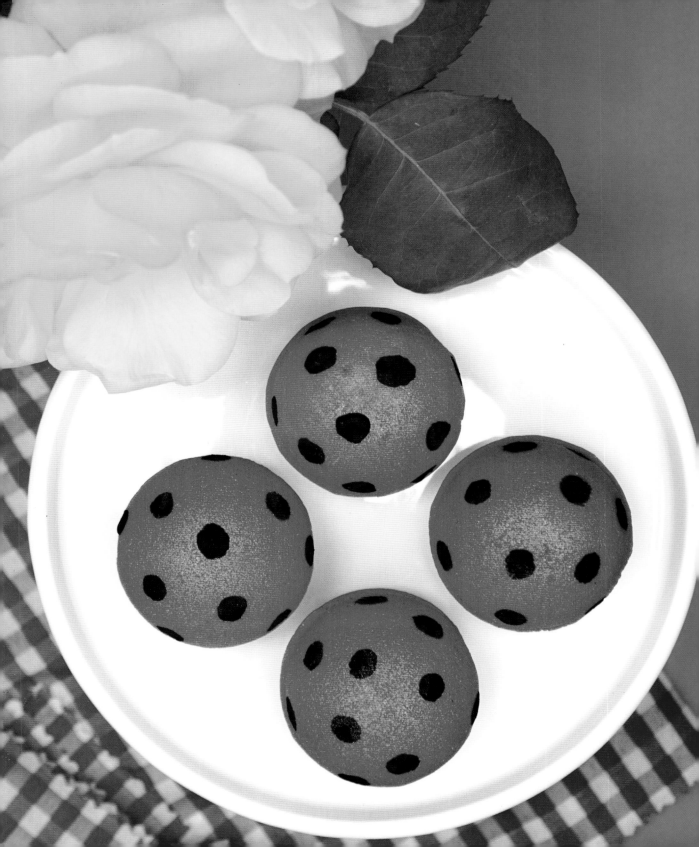

LADYBUG
BATH BOMBS

For a splash of good luck, add lovely ladybugs to your bath time. Let the aromatic scent of roses whisk you away to the garden and release your stresses as you bathe in rose-colored water and velvety soft suds. You're guaranteed to feel fortunate as you soak!

MAKES

7

BATH BOMBS

SUPPLIES

1½ cups baking soda

1½ tablespoons cream of tartar

1½ tablespoons white kaolin clay

1½ tablespoons sodium lauryl sulfoacetate (SLSA)

1 teaspoon red mica colorant

1 tablespoon sweet almond oil

½ tablespoon polysorbate 80

15 drops rose essential oil

¼ teaspoon water

¾ cup citric acid

Witch hazel, scant amount as needed

2″ round bath bomb mold

½ teaspoon isopropyl alcohol

¼ teaspoon activated charcoal powder

MIXING DIRECTIONS

1 · In a large mixing bowl, thoroughly combine the baking soda, cream of tartar, kaolin clay, SLSA, and red mica.

2 · In a small container, stir together the sweet almond oil, polysorbate 80, rose essential oil, and water. Stirring constantly, slowly add the liquids into the dry ingredients until they are completely combined.

3 · Add the citric acid to the mixture and stir until it is fully incorporated. If the mixture is not quite wet enough to mold, spritz two to three times with a spray bottle of witch hazel and mix well. Repeat as necessary.

MOLDING DIRECTIONS

4 · Lightly overfill both halves of the mold with the mixture. Press the halves firmly together.

5 · Carefully release the bath bomb from the mold and allow it to dry completely for 24–48 hours. Repeat to create the remaining bath bombs.

6 · In a small container, mix together the isopropyl alcohol and activated charcoal powder. Use a paintbrush to apply black polka dots to the bath bombs.

STARFISH & SEASHELL
BATH BOMBS

et the ocean breeze fragrance whisk you away to sandy beaches and sunny shores as you bathe in softly colored water with a shimmery layer of fizz. Rich mango butter in these bath bombs will leave your skin silky smooth and supple.

MAKES

5 and **10**

STARFISH   SEASHELL

BATH BOMBS

SUPPLIES

4 cups baking soda

½ cup cornstarch

2 tablespoons cream of tartar

2 tablespoons white kaolin clay

2 tablespoons sodium lauryl sulfoacetate (SLSA)

½ teaspoon orange mica colorant

½ teaspoon pink mica colorant

½ teaspoon lilac mica colorant

2 tablespoons coconut oil, melted and divided

2 tablespoons mango butter, melted and divided

1 tablespoon polysorbate 80, divided

1 teaspoon awapuhi seaberry fragrance oil, divided

2 cups citric acid, divided

Witch hazel, scant amount as needed

Gold and iridescent cosmetic glitter

Metal starfish and seashell bath bomb molds

MIXING DIRECTIONS

1 · In a large mixing bowl, thoroughly combine the baking soda, cornstarch, cream of tartar, kaolin clay, and SLSA. Divide the mixture evenly into four medium bowls. Mix the orange mica into one bowl, the pink into the second bowl, the lilac into the third bowl, and leave the fourth bowl uncolored.

2 · In a small container, combine ½ tablespoon of the melted coconut oil, ½ tablespoon of the melted mango butter, ¼ tablespoon of the polysorbate 80, and ¼ teaspoon of the awapuhi seaberry fragrance oil. Stirring constantly, slowly mix the liquids into the orange dry ingredients until they are completely combined. Repeat this step for each of the different colored bowls.

$3 \cdot$ Add ½ cup of the citric acid to each of the bowls and stir until it is fully incorporated into the mixture. If the mixture is not quite wet enough to mold, spritz two to three times with a spray bottle of witch hazel and mix well. Repeat as necessary.

MOLDING DIRECTIONS

$4 \cdot$ Press the bath bomb mixture firmly into the molds using your thumb and the palm of your hand to apply pressure. Fill the molds to the top until they are packed completely full.

$5 \cdot$ Carefully release the bath bombs from the molds and allow them to dry completely for 24–48 hours. When the bath bombs are dry, dust the surface with cosmetic glitter for extra sparkle and shimmer.

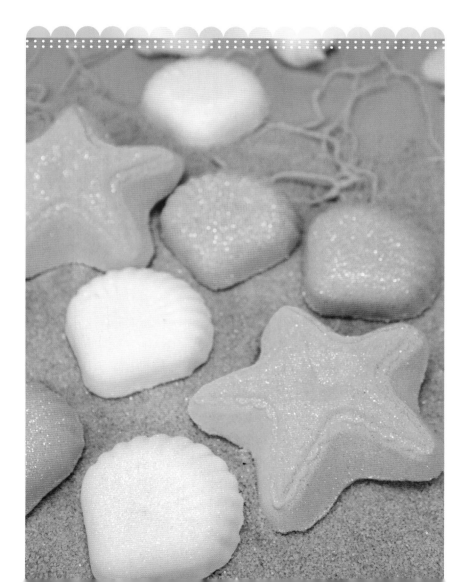

EARTH
BATH BOMBS

Take a trip around the world in your very own bathtub with these amazing Earth bath bombs! Calm your body and mind as you sink into an aromatic aqua-colored pool of silky suds that will nourish your skin and rejuvenate your spirit.

MAKES

BATH BOMBS

SUPPLIES

3 cups baking soda

2 tablespoons cream of tartar

⅓ cup cornstarch

2 tablespoons sodium lauryl sulfoacetate (SLSA)

1 teaspoon blue mica colorant

1 teaspoon green mica colorant

2 tablespoons avocado oil, divided

1 tablespoon polysorbate 80, divided

½ teaspoon mountain rain fragrance oil

½ teaspoon bamboo fragrance oil

1½ cups citric acid, divided

Witch hazel, scant amount as needed

2½" round bath bomb mold

MIXING DIRECTIONS

1 · In a large mixing bowl, thoroughly combine the baking soda, cream of tartar, cornstarch, and SLSA. Divide the mixture evenly into two medium bowls. Mix the blue mica into one bowl and the green mica into the second bowl.

2 · In a small container, combine 1 tablespoon of the avocado oil, ½ tablespoon of the polysorbate 80, and the mountain rain fragrance oil. Stirring constantly, slowly mix the liquids into the blue dry ingredients until they are completely combined.

3 · In another small container, combine the remaining avocado oil and polysorbate 80 and the bamboo fragrance oil. Stirring constantly, slowly mix the liquids into the green dry ingredients until they are completely combined.

4 · Add ¾ cup of the citric acid to each of the bowls and stir until it is fully incorporated into the mixture. If the mixture is not quite wet enough to mold, spritz two to three times with a spray bottle of witch hazel and mix well. Repeat as necessary.

MOLDING DIRECTIONS

5 · Fill both halves of the mold with varied sections of blue and green bath bomb mixture. Make sure to overfill the mold just a bit. Press the halves firmly together.

6 · Carefully release the bath bomb from the mold and allow it to dry completely for 24–48 hours. Repeat to create the remaining bath bombs.

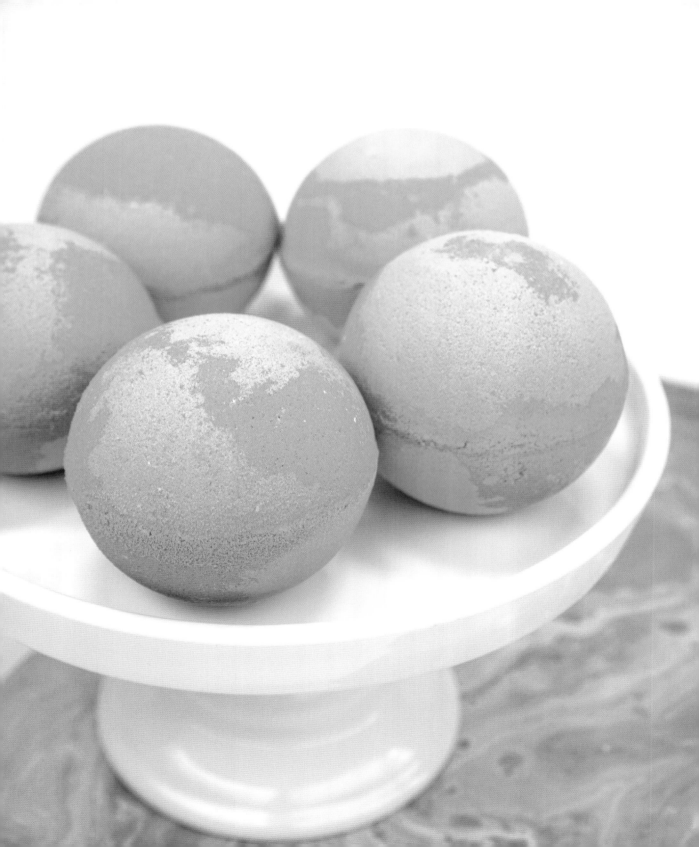

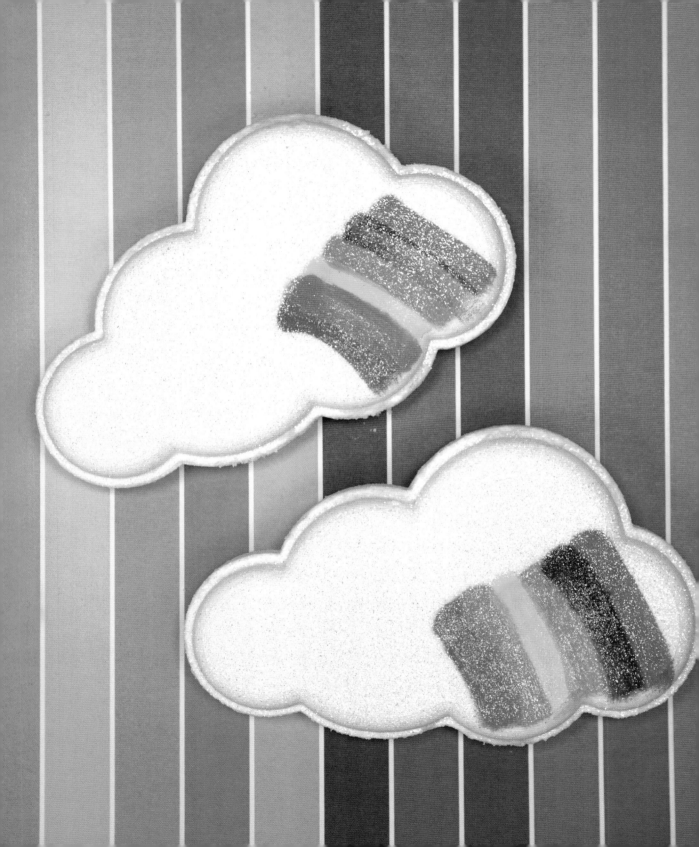

RAINBOW CLOUD
BATH BOMBS

Everyone loves a fun surprise, and these sparkly clouds are hiding a rainbow-colored secret inside! Colorful bath bomb embeds will release a rainbow of concentrated color as the bath bomb fizzes and fills your bathtub with brightly colored swirls of foam and bubbles.

MAKES

BATH BOMBS

SUPPLIES

3 cups baking soda

½ cup cornstarch

2 tablespoons cream of tartar

2 tablespoons kaolin clay

2½ tablespoons sodium
   lauryl sulfoacetate (SLSA)

2 tablespoons sweet almond oil

1 tablespoon polysorbate 80

1 teaspoon rain fragrance oil

½ teaspoon water

1½ cups citric acid

Witch hazel, scant
   amount as needed

Bath bomb embeds in a
   rainbow of colors

3 teaspoons isopropyl alcohol

¼ teaspoon each mica colorant
   in red, orange, yellow,
   green, blue, and purple

Iridescent cosmetic glitter

3-piece cloud bath bomb mold

MIXING DIRECTIONS

1 · In a large mixing bowl, thoroughly combine the baking soda, cornstarch, cream of tartar, kaolin clay, and SLSA.

2 · In a small container, stir together the sweet almond oil, polysorbate 80, rain fragrance oil, and water. Stirring constantly, slowly add the liquids into the dry ingredients until they are completely combined.

3 · Add the citric acid to the mixture and stir until it is fully incorporated. If the mixture is not quite wet enough to mold, spritz two to three times with a spray bottle of witch hazel and mix well. Repeat as necessary.

MOLDING DIRECTIONS

4 · Place the bottom half of the mold inside the molding ring. Loosely pack the bath bomb mixture inside the bottom half of the mold. Add the colored embeds inside the middle of the bath bomb and continue to fill the remainder of the mold, overfilling just slightly. Press the top half of the mold firmly into the ring. Flip the mold over and press again from the opposite side. Slide the ring off the mold and carefully unmold the bath bomb. Allow to dry completely for 24-48 hours. Repeat to create the remaining bath bombs.

5 · When the bath bombs are dry, dust them with iridescent cosmetic glitter. Combine ½ teaspoon of the isopropyl alcohol with ¼ teaspoon of each mica colorant and use a paintbrush to apply rainbow mica stripes to the cloud.

GALAXY
BATH BOMBS

These bath bombs deliver an out-of-this-world bath-time experience! Activated charcoal gently cleanses skin by drawing out dirt, chemicals, and bacteria, while coconut oil and aloe butter deliver exceptional hydration to leave you feeling purified and refreshed.

MAKES

10

BATH BOMBS

SUPPLIES

1½ cups baking soda

½ cup Epsom salt, finely ground

2 tablespoons arrowroot powder

1 tablespoon sodium lauryl sulfoacetate (SLSA)

1 tablespoon activated charcoal powder

1 tablespoon fractionated coconut oil

1 tablespoon aloe butter, melted

1 tablespoon polysorbate 80

½ teaspoon night air fragrance oil

¾ cup citric acid

Witch hazel, scant amount as needed

Hard plastic bath bomb mold

1½ teaspoons isopropyl alcohol, divided

¼ teaspoon midnight blue mica

¼ teaspoon purple mica

¼ teaspoon light gold mica

MIXING DIRECTIONS

1· In a large mixing bowl, thoroughly combine the baking soda, Epsom salt, arrowroot powder, SLSA, and activated charcoal powder.

2· In a small container, mix together the fractionated coconut oil, melted aloe butter, polysorbate 80, and night air fragrance oil. Stirring constantly, slowly mix the liquids into the dry ingredients until they are completely combined.

3· Add the citric acid to the mixture and stir until it is fully incorporated. If the mixture is not quite wet enough to mold, spritz two to three times with a spray bottle of witch hazel and mix well. Repeat as necessary.

MOLDING DIRECTIONS

4· Press the bath bomb mixture firmly into the mold using your thumb and the palm of your hand to apply pressure. Fill the mold to the top until it is packed completely full.

5· Carefully release the bath bomb from the mold and allow it to dry completely for 24–48 hours. Repeat to create the remaining bath bombs.

6· When the bath bombs are dry, mix ½ teaspoon of isopropyl alcohol with each of the three mica powders: light gold, midnight blue, and purple. Use a stiff paintbrush to splatter paint the bath bombs with midnight blue and purple; let dry. Then use a soft paintbrush to add gold star details.

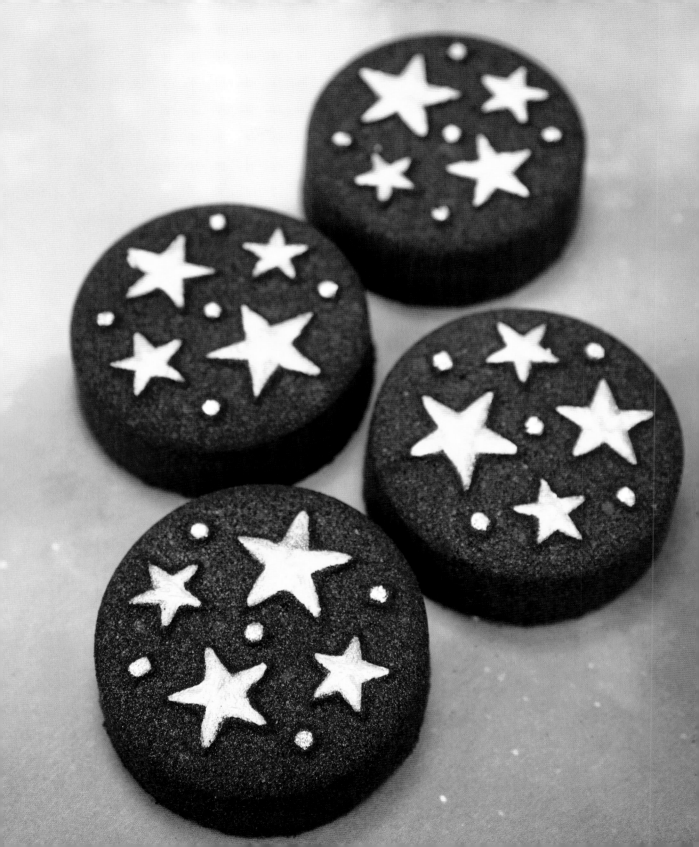

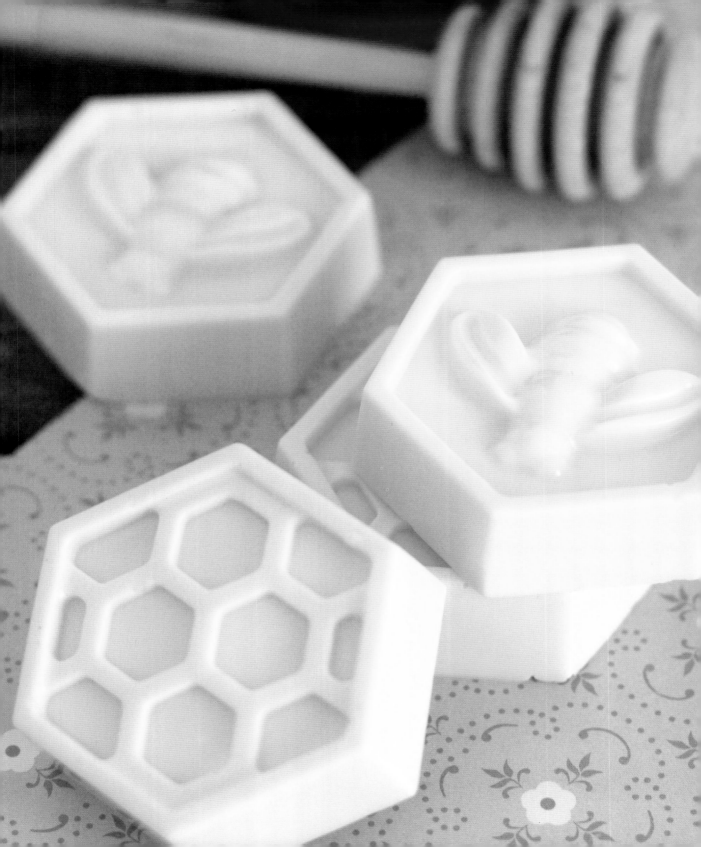

MILK & HONEY
SOAPS

These soaps not only smell amazing but also boast lots of healthy skin benefits! Goat's milk is a wonderful moisturizer, and honey is clarifying, soothing, and naturally antibacterial. The combination can fight acne and signs of aging and brighten your skin.

MAKES

19

SOAPS

SUPPLIES

2 pounds goat's milk soap base

Microwave-safe measuring cup

6 drops gold soap colorant

5 tablespoons raw honey

10 drops honeysuckle
  fragrance oil, optional

Isopropyl alcohol, in
  a spray bottle

12″ silicone honeycomb mold

DIRECTIONS

1 · Slice the goat's milk soap base into small cubes and place into a microwave-safe measuring cup. Melt in the microwave in 30-second increments, stirring well after each session to ensure that the soap is completely melted.

2 · Carefully stir in the gold soap colorant and honey. If you find that your honey doesn't give the soap enough scent, you may also wish to add 10 drops of honeysuckle fragrance oil. Pour the melted soap into the mold and spritz with isopropyl alcohol to remove any air bubbles.

3 · Allow the soaps to sit undisturbed until completely firm (approximately 60–90 minutes depending on temperature and humidity) before unmolding.

SNOWFLAKE
SUGAR SCRUB BARS

These sugar scrub bars gently exfoliate for unbelievably smooth skin. Rich coconut oil and fine grains of sugar combine with sumptuous shea butter soap for a skin-rejuvenating experience.

MAKES

12

SUGAR SCRUB BARS

SUPPLIES

2 pounds shea butter soap base

Microwave-safe measuring cup

6 drops blue soap colorant

2 cups granulated sugar, divided

6 tablespoons coconut oil, melted and divided

1 teaspoon iridescent cosmetic glitter, divided

1 teaspoon pearl shimmer mica powder, divided

Isopropyl alcohol, in a spray bottle

Silicone snowflake mold

DIRECTIONS

1 · Slice the shea butter soap base into small cubes and divide into two piles. Place the first half of the cubes into a microwave-safe measuring cup. Melt in the microwave in 30-second increments, stirring well after each session to ensure that the soap is completely melted.

2 · Carefully stir in the blue soap colorant, 1 cup of the granulated sugar, 3 tablespoons of the melted coconut oil, ½ teaspoon of the iridescent cosmetic glitter, and ½ teaspoon of the pearl shimmer mica. Pour the liquid mixture into the mold and spritz with isopropyl alcohol to remove any air bubbles.

3 · Allow the sugar scrub bars to sit undisturbed until completely firm (approximately 60–90 minutes depending on temperature and humidity) before unmolding.

4 · Repeat the process with the other half of the soap base cubes and remaining ingredients, omitting the blue soap colorant, to make white sugar scrub snowflakes.

·CHAPTER FOUR·

COLOR &

SPARKLE

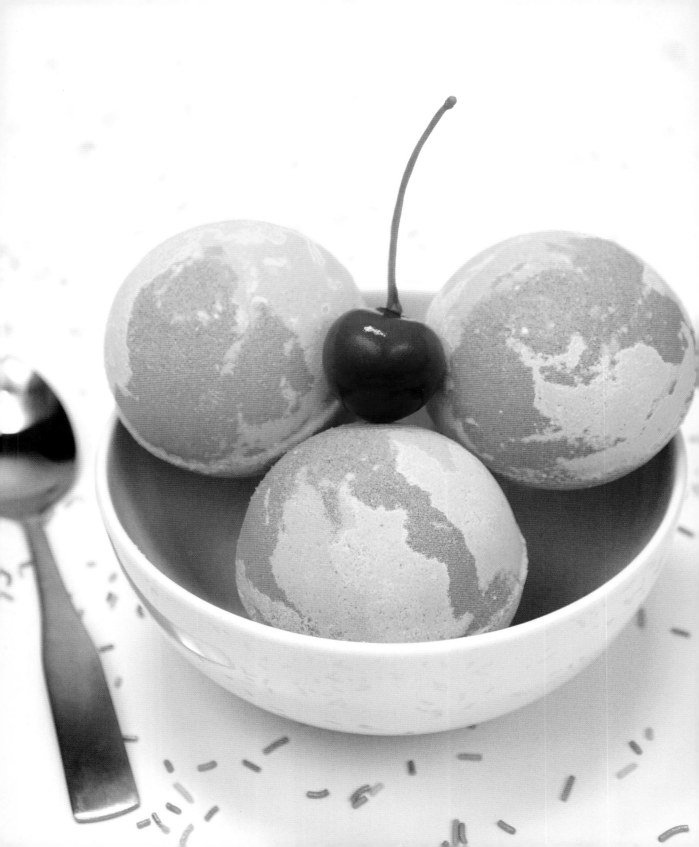

RAINBOW SHERBET
BATH BOMBS

These bath bombs are a colorful delight. Fill your bathtub with the fruity fragrances of raspberry, orange, and lime and a helping of coconut oil that will leave your skin glowing and smelling sweet.

MAKES

BATH BOMBS

SUPPLIES

3 cups baking soda

½ cup cornstarch

½ cup Epsom salt, finely ground

2 tablespoons cream of tartar

1 tablespoon sodium lauryl sulfoacetate (SLSA)

1 teaspoon pink mica colorant

1 teaspoon orange mica colorant

1 teaspoon neon green mica colorant

3 tablespoons coconut oil, melted

1½ tablespoons polysorbate 80, divided

25 drops orange essential oil

25 drops lime essential oil

½ teaspoon raspberry fragrance oil

1½ cups citric acid, divided

Witch hazel, scant amount as needed

2½″ round bath bomb mold

Chopstick or similar item

MIXING DIRECTIONS

1 · In a large mixing bowl, thoroughly combine the baking soda, cornstarch, Epsom salt, cream of tartar, and SLSA. Divide the mixture evenly into three medium bowls. Mix the pink mica into one bowl, the orange into the second bowl, and the neon green into the third.

2 · In a small container, combine 1 tablespoon of the melted coconut oil, ½ tablespoon of the polysorbate 80, and the raspberry fragrance oil. Stirring constantly, slowly mix the liquids into the pink dry ingredients until they are completely combined.

3 · In another small container, combine 1 tablespoon of the melted coconut oil, ½ tablespoon of the polysorbate 80, and the orange essential oil. Stirring constantly, slowly mix the liquids into the orange dry ingredients until they are completely combined.

4 · In a third small container, combine the remaining melted coconut oil and polysorbate 80 with the lime essential oil. Stirring constantly, slowly mix the liquids into the neon green dry ingredients until they are completely combined.

5 · Stir ½ cup of the citric acid into each of the bowls. If the mixture is not quite wet enough to mold, spritz two to three times with a spray bottle of witch hazel and mix well. Repeat as necessary.

MOLDING DIRECTIONS

6 · Lightly overfill both halves of the mold with the colored mixtures and swirl with a chopstick. Press the halves firmly together.

7 · Carefully release the bath bomb from the mold and allow it to dry completely for 24–48 hours. Repeat to create the remaining bath bombs.

MERMAID
BATH BOMBS

Transform bath time into a captivating under-the-sea experience with these whimsical mermaid bath bombs! Let the scents of the ocean carry you away to a land of carefree bliss as you catch a wave of shimmery, colorful bubbles and relax in a pool of deep blue.

MAKES

BATH BOMBS

SUPPLIES

3 cups baking soda

1½ tablespoons cream of tartar

2 tablespoons sodium lauryl sulfoacetate (SLSA)

1 teaspoon turquoise mica colorant

1 teaspoon purple mica colorant

2 tablespoons fractionated coconut oil, divided

1 tablespoon polysorbate 80, divided

1 teaspoon cocamidopropyl betaine

½ teaspoon ocean breeze fragrance oil

½ teaspoon sun and sand fragrance oil

1½ cups citric acid, divided

Witch hazel, scant amount as needed

Iridescent cosmetic glitter

2½" round bath bomb mold

MIXING DIRECTIONS

1· In a large mixing bowl, thoroughly combine the baking soda, cream of tartar, and SLSA. Divide the mixture evenly into two medium bowls. Mix the turquoise mica into one bowl and the purple mica into the second bowl.

2· In a small container, combine 1 tablespoon of the fractionated coconut oil, ½ tablespoon of the polysorbate 80, ½ teaspoon of the cocamidopropyl betaine, and the ocean breeze fragrance oil. Stirring constantly, slowly mix the liquids into the turquoise dry ingredients until they are completely combined.

$3\cdot$ In another small container, combine the remaining fractionated coconut oil, polysorbate 80, cocamidopropyl betaine, and the sun and sand fragrance oil. Stirring constantly, slowly mix the liquids into the purple dry ingredients until they are completely combined.

$4\cdot$ Add ¾ cup of the citric acid to each of the bowls and stir until it is fully incorporated into the mixture. If the mixture is not quite wet enough to mold, spritz two to three times with a spray bottle of witch hazel and mix well. Repeat as necessary.

MOLDING DIRECTIONS

$5\cdot$ Fill the mold with freeform stripes of turquoise and purple bath bomb mixture. Make sure to overfill the mold just a bit. Press the halves firmly together.

$6\cdot$ Carefully release the bath bomb from the mold and allow it to dry completely for 24–48 hours. Repeat to create the remaining bath bombs.

$7\cdot$ When the bath bombs are dry, brush with iridescent cosmetic glitter to add sparkle and shimmer.

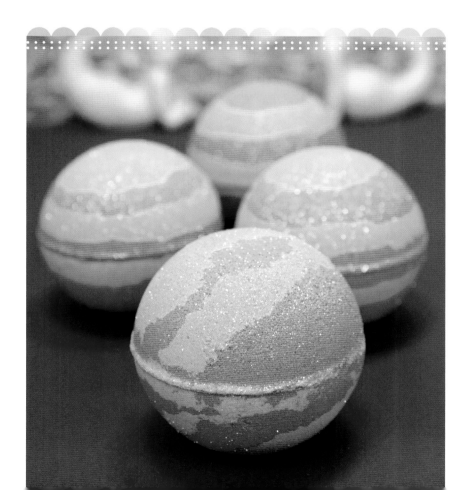

UNICORN
BATH BOMBS

Shimmery, hand-painted details make these unicorn bath bombs truly shine. Envision dreams coming true as layers of softly colored foam and sparkle appear. Shea butter will soothe and revitalize your skin for pure bath-time magic.

MAKES

12

BATH BOMBS

SUPPLIES

3 cups baking soda

½ cup cornstarch

½ cup Epsom salt, finely ground

2 tablespoons white kaolin clay

2 tablespoons sodium lauryl sulfoacetate (SLSA)

2 tablespoons sweet almond oil

2 tablespoons shea butter, melted

½ tablespoon polysorbate 80

1 teaspoon bubble gum fragrance oil

½ teaspoon water

1½ cup citric acid

Witch hazel, scant amount as needed

Hard plastic unicorn bath bomb mold

Iridescent cosmetic glitter

2¼ teaspoons isopropyl alcohol, divided

⅛ teaspoon activated charcoal powder

¼ teaspoon gold mica colorant

¼ teaspoon purple mica colorant

¼ teaspoon magenta mica colorant

¼ teaspoon teal mica colorant

Gold cosmetic glitter

MIXING DIRECTIONS

1· In a large mixing bowl, thoroughly combine the baking soda, cornstarch, Epsom salt, kaolin clay, and SLSA.

2· In a small container, mix together the sweet almond oil, melted shea butter, polysorbate 80, bubble gum fragrance oil, and water. Stirring constantly, slowly mix the liquids into the dry ingredients until they are completely combined.

$3 \cdot$ Add the citric acid to the mixture and stir until it is fully incorporated. If the mixture is not quite wet enough to mold, spritz two to three times with a spray bottle of witch hazel and mix well. Repeat as necessary.

MOLDING DIRECTIONS

$4 \cdot$ Press the bath bomb mixture firmly into the mold using your thumb and the palm of your hand to apply pressure. Fill the mold to the top until it is packed completely full.

$5 \cdot$ Carefully release the bath bomb from the mold and allow it to dry completely for 24–48 hours. Repeat to create the remaining bath bombs.

$6 \cdot$ When dry, brush the bath bombs with a layer of iridescent cosmetic glitter. Mix the activated charcoal with ¼ teaspoon of the isopropyl alcohol and use a paintbrush to add the unicorn's eye details. Mix ½ teaspoon of the isopropyl alcohol with each of the gold, purple, magenta, and teal micas. Use a paintbrush to add horn and mane details and add gold cosmetic glitter to the horn.

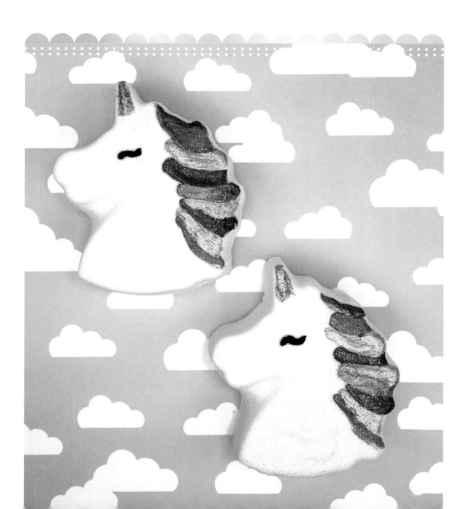

RAINBOW STRIPED
BATH BOMBS

These stunning bath bombs fill your tub with loads of fluffy bubbles and sweet-scented fizz. Your skin will feel sleek and smooth thanks to the addition of shea butter and sweet almond oil. This recipe makes an extra-large batch of bath bombs, but they are worth the effort!

MAKES

18

BATH BOMBS

SUPPLIES

12 cups baking soda

2 cups Epsom salt, finely ground

1½ cups cornstarch

½ cup cream of tartar

½ cup white kaolin clay

½ cup sodium lauryl sulfoacetate (SLSA)

1 teaspoon each mica colorant in red, orange, yellow, green, blue, and purple

½ cup + 1 tablespoon sweet almond oil, divided

½ cup + 1 tablespoon shea butter, melted and divided

3 teaspoons cocamidopropyl betaine, divided

3 tablespoons polysorbate 80, divided

3 teaspoons fruit cereal fragrance oil, divided

6 cups citric acid, divided

Witch hazel, scant amount as needed

3" round bath bomb mold

MIXING DIRECTIONS

1 · In an extra-large mixing bowl, thoroughly combine the baking soda, Epsom salt, cornstarch, cream of tartar, kaolin clay, and SLSA. Divide the mixture evenly into six bowls and color each bowl with the red, orange, yellow, green, blue, and purple mica.

2 · In a small container, mix together 1½ tablespoons of the sweet almond oil, 1½ tablespoons of the melted shea butter, ½ teaspoon of the cocamidopropyl betaine, ½ tablespoon of the polysorbate 80, and ½ teaspoon of the fruit cereal fragrance oil. Stirring constantly, slowly mix the liquids into the red dry ingredients until they are completely combined. Repeat the process for all the other colored mixtures.

3 · Add 1 cup of the citric acid to the each of the different colored bowls and stir until it is fully incorporated. If the mixture is not quite wet enough to mold, spritz two to three times with a spray bottle of witch hazel and mix well. Repeat as necessary.

MOLDING DIRECTIONS

4 · Layer the colored mixtures into both halves of the mold in a striped pattern. Make sure to overfill the mold just a bit. Press the halves firmly together.

5 · Carefully release the bath bomb from the mold and allow it to dry completely for 24–48 hours. Repeat to create the remaining bath bombs.

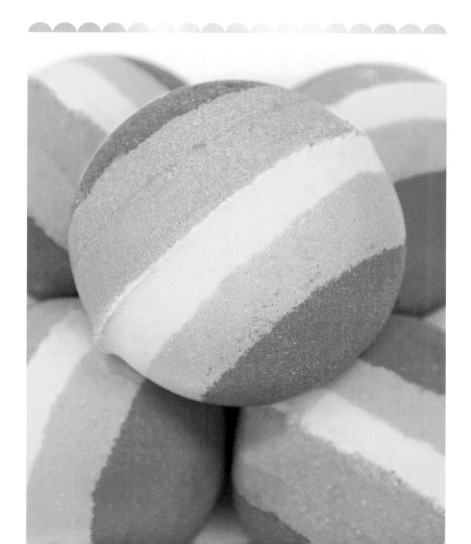

STARRY NIGHT
BATH BOMBS

Reminiscent of Van Gogh's famous swirls and colors, these Starry Night-inspired bath bombs are a dream in your tub! Drift into a place of peace as you relax in the aqua water and take in the juniper breeze fragrance.

MAKES

12

BATH BOMBS

SUPPLIES

4 cups baking soda

½ cup cornstarch

½ cup Epsom salt, finely ground

2 tablespoons cream of tartar

2 tablespoons sodium lauryl
    sulfoacetate (SLSA)

1 teaspoon dark blue
    mica colorant

½ teaspoon light blue
    mica colorant

½ teaspoon yellow
    mica colorant

2 tablespoons fractionated
    coconut oil, divided

2 tablespoons polysorbate
    80, divided

1 tablespoon juniper breeze
    fragrance oil, divided

2 cups citric acid, divided

Witch hazel, scant
    amount as needed

2½″ round bath bomb mold

Chopstick or similar item

MIXING DIRECTIONS

1 · In a large mixing bowl, thoroughly combine the baking soda, cornstarch, Epsom salt, cream of tartar, and SLSA. Separate the mixture into three medium-sized bowls—half of the mixture into the first bowl, and a quarter of the mixture into the other two bowls. Mix the dark blue mica into the first bowl and the yellow mica into the second bowl. In the third bowl, loosely mix the light blue mica into the white so that there are areas of both light blue and white in the mixture.

2 · In a small container, combine 1 tablespoon of the fractionated coconut oil, 1 tablespoon of the polysorbate 80, and ½ tablespoon of the juniper breeze fragrance oil. Stirring constantly, slowly mix the liquids into the dark blue dry ingredients until they are completely combined.

3 · In another small container, combine ½ tablespoon of the fractionated coconut oil, ½ tablespoon of the polysorbate 80, and ¼ tablespoon of the juniper breeze fragrance oil. Stirring constantly, slowly mix the liquids into the yellow dry ingredients until they are completely combined.

4 · In a third small container, combine the remaining ½ tablespoon of fractionated coconut oil, ½ tablespoon of polysorbate 80, and ¼ tablespoon of juniper breeze fragrance oil. Stirring constantly, slowly mix the liquids into the light blue dry ingredients until they are completely combined.

5 · Add 1 cup of the citric acid to the dark blue mixture and stir until it is fully incorporated. Add ½ cup of the citric acid each to the yellow and light blue mixtures and stir until thoroughly mixed. If the mixture is not quite wet enough to mold, spritz two to three times with a spray bottle of witch hazel and mix well. Repeat as necessary.

MOLDING DIRECTIONS

6 · Fill both halves of the mold with alternating areas of dark blue (primarily), light blue, and yellow. Use a chopstick to swirl the colors inside each half of the mold. Make sure to overfill both sides of the mold just a bit. Press the halves firmly together.

7 · Carefully release the bath bomb from the mold and allow it to dry completely for 24–48 hours. Repeat to create the remaining bath bombs.

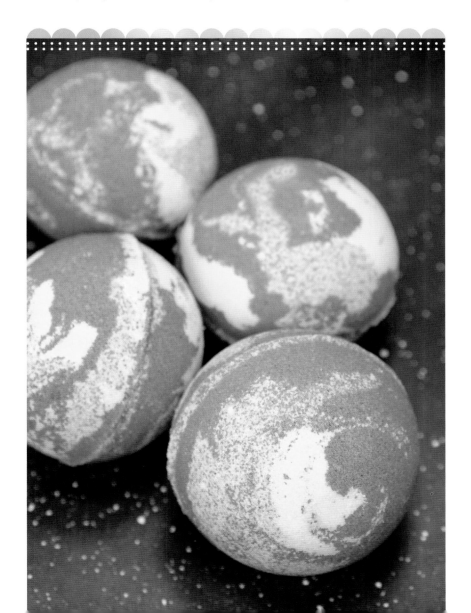

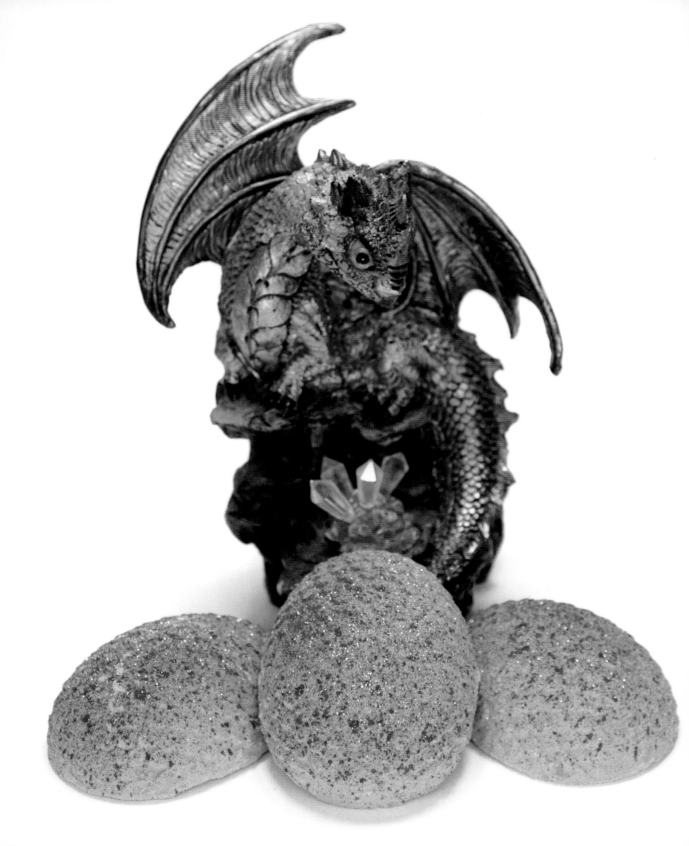

DRAGON'S EGG
BATH BOMBS

Mystical dragon's egg bath bombs are an enchanting way to relax. Soak the stresses of the day away among swells of bubbles in sky-colored water with a hint of shimmer. Rich argan oil, known for its smoothing and hydrating properties, will leave your skin magically soft.

MAKES

5

BATH BOMBS

SUPPLIES

1½ cups baking soda

1½ tablespoons cream of tartar

3 tablespoons cornstarch

2 tablespoons sodium lauryl sulfoacetate (SLSA)

½ teaspoon blue mica colorant

1½ tablespoons argan oil

½ tablespoon polysorbate 80, divided

1 teaspoon cocamidopropyl betaine

½ teaspoon dragon's blood fragrance oil

¾ cup citric acid, divided

Witch hazel, scant amount as needed

Hard plastic dragon egg mold

½ teaspoon isopropyl alcohol

¼ teaspoon purple mica colorant

Blue iridescent cosmetic glitter

MIXING DIRECTIONS

1 · In a large mixing bowl, thoroughly combine the baking soda, cream of tartar, cornstarch, SLSA, and blue mica.

2 · In a small container, combine the argan oil, polysorbate 80, cocamidopropyl betaine, and dragon's blood fragrance oil. Stirring constantly, slowly mix the liquids into the dry ingredients until they are completely combined.

3 · Add the citric acid and stir until it is fully incorporated into the mixture. If the mixture is not quite wet enough to mold, spritz two to three times with a spray bottle of witch hazel and mix well. Repeat as necessary.

MOLDING DIRECTIONS

4 · Press the bath bomb mixture firmly into the mold using your thumb and the palm of your hand to apply pressure. Fill the mold to the top until it is packed completely full.

5 · Carefully release the bath bombs from the mold and allow to dry completely for 24–48 hours. Repeat to create the remaining bath bombs.

6 · Once dry, mix the isopropyl alcohol and purple mica and use a stiff paintbrush to splatter the bath bombs. Use a soft paintbrush to dust on a layer of blue iridescent cosmetic glitter.

SURPRISE INSIDE
BATH BOMBS

These sweetly scented bath bombs are hiding a super secret. Each colorful, fizzy bath bomb has a treasure tucked inside to make bath time even more delightful. Have fun selecting just what the prizes will be!

MAKES

10

BATH BOMBS

SUPPLIES

3 cups baking soda

1½ tablespoons cream of tartar

2 tablespoons white kaolin clay

2 tablespoons sodium lauryl sulfoacetate (SLSA)

½ teaspoon pink mica colorant

½ teaspoon purple mica colorant

2 tablespoons apricot kernel oil, divided

1 tablespoon polysorbate 80, divided

1 teaspoon cocamidopropyl betaine, divided

1 teaspoon bubble gum fragrance oil, divided

1½ cups citric acid, divided

Witch hazel, scant amount as needed

2½" round bath bomb mold

Chopstick or similar item

10 mini plastic capsules (approximately 1⅛") filled with jewelry or small trinkets

MIXING DIRECTIONS

1 · In a large mixing bowl, thoroughly combine the baking soda, cream of tartar, kaolin clay, and SLSA. Divide the mixture evenly into two medium bowls. Mix the pink mica into one bowl and the purple mica into the second bowl.

2 · In a small container, combine 1 tablespoon of the apricot kernel oil, ½ tablespoon of the polysorbate 80, ½ teaspoon of the cocamidopropyl betaine, and ½ teaspoon of the bubble gum fragrance oil. Stirring constantly, slowly mix the liquids into the pink dry ingredients until they are completely combined.

3 · In another small container, combine the remaining apricot kernel oil, polysorbate 80, cocamidopropyl betaine, and bubble gum fragrance oil. Stirring constantly, slowly mix the liquids into the purple dry ingredients until they are completely combined.

4 · Stir ¾ cup of the citric acid into each of the bowls. If the mixture is not quite wet enough to mold, spritz two to three times with a spray bottle of witch hazel and mix well. Repeat as necessary.

MOLDING DIRECTIONS

5 · Fill half of the mold with small random areas of the pink and purple bath bomb mixtures. Use a chopstick to swirl the colors together. Place a filled capsule into the center of the first half of the mold. Fill the second half of the mold, swirling the two colors with a chopstick. Make sure to overfill the mold just a bit. Press the halves firmly together.

6 · Carefully release the bath bomb from the mold and allow it to dry completely for 24–48 hours. Repeat to create the remaining bath bombs.

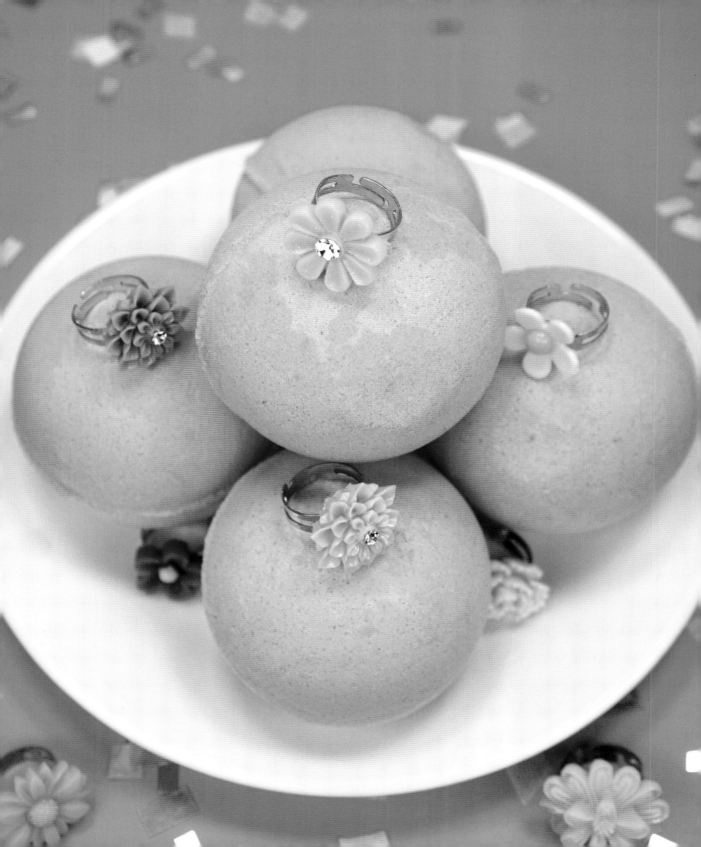

JEWEL
BATH BOMBS

Invite riches into your home with these elegant jewel bath bombs! Sweet orange and patchouli oils have long been thought to attract wealth and abundance. Even if you don't believe the legends, these shimmery jewels are surely rich in moisturizers and sparkly foam.

MAKES

10

BATH BOMBS

SUPPLIES

1½ cups baking soda

1 tablespoon cream of tartar

1 tablespoon sodium lauryl sulfoacetate (SLSA)

1 tablespoon jojoba oil

½ tablespoon polysorbate 80

25 drops sweet orange essential oil

10 drops patchouli essential oil

¾ cup citric acid

Witch hazel, scant amount as needed

¼ teaspoon mica colorant in red, orange, yellow, green, blue, and purple

3 teaspoons isopropyl alcohol, divided

Assorted cosmetic glitters

Gemstone mold

MIXING DIRECTIONS

1 · In a large mixing bowl, thoroughly combine the baking soda, cream of tartar, and SLSA.

2 · In a small container, mix together the jojoba oil, polysorbate 80, sweet orange essential oil, and patchouli essential oil. Stirring constantly, slowly mix the liquids into the dry ingredients until they are completely combined.

3 · Add the citric acid to the mixture and stir until it is fully incorporated. If the mixture is not quite wet enough to mold, spritz two to three times with a spray bottle of witch hazel and mix well. Repeat as necessary.

MOLDING DIRECTIONS

4 · Press the bath bomb mixture firmly into the mold using your thumb and the palm of your hand to apply pressure. Fill the mold to the top until it is packed completely full.

5 · Carefully release the bath bombs from the mold and allow them to dry completely for 24–48 hours.

6 · When the bath bombs are dry, mix ¼ teaspoon of each mica colorant with ½ teaspoon of the isopropyl alcohol, and use a paintbrush to add color to each gemstone. Alternately, you can also mix the mica and alcohol in a spray bottle and spray the gemstones with color. Finish with a layer of cosmetic glitter to match the color of the gemstone.

HIDDEN COLOR
BATH BOMBS

These unassuming white bath bombs may look plain and simple, but they're packed full of intense color! Fill the center of each bath bomb with highly pigmented embeds for a surprise explosion of color and fizz when they hit the water.

MAKES

10

BATH BOMBS

SUPPLIES

3 cups baking soda

½ cup Epsom salt, finely ground

½ cup cornstarch

2 tablespoons white kaolin clay

1 tablespoon arrowroot powder

2 tablespoons sodium lauryl
   sulfoacetate (SLSA)

2 tablespoons sweet almond oil

1 tablespoon mango
   butter, melted

1 tablespoon polysorbate 80

1 teaspoon peaches and
   cream fragrance oil

½ teaspoon water

1½ cups citric acid

Witch hazel, scant
   amount as needed

2½" round bath bomb mold

Colored embeds

MIXING DIRECTIONS

1 · In a large mixing bowl, thoroughly combine the baking soda, Epsom salt, cornstarch, kaolin clay, arrowroot powder, and SLSA.

2 · In a small container, mix together the sweet almond oil, melted mango butter, polysorbate 80, peaches and cream fragrance oil, and water. Stirring constantly, slowly mix the liquids into the dry ingredients until they are completely combined.

3 · Add the citric acid to the mixture and stir until it is fully incorporated. If the mixture is not quite wet enough to mold, spritz two to three times with a spray bottle of witch hazel and mix well. Repeat as necessary.

MOLDING DIRECTIONS

4 · Lightly overfill both halves of the mold with the mixture and place colorful embeds inside of one half of the mold. Press the halves firmly together.

5 · Carefully release the bath bomb from the mold and allow it to dry completely for 24–48 hours. Repeat to create the remaining bath bombs.

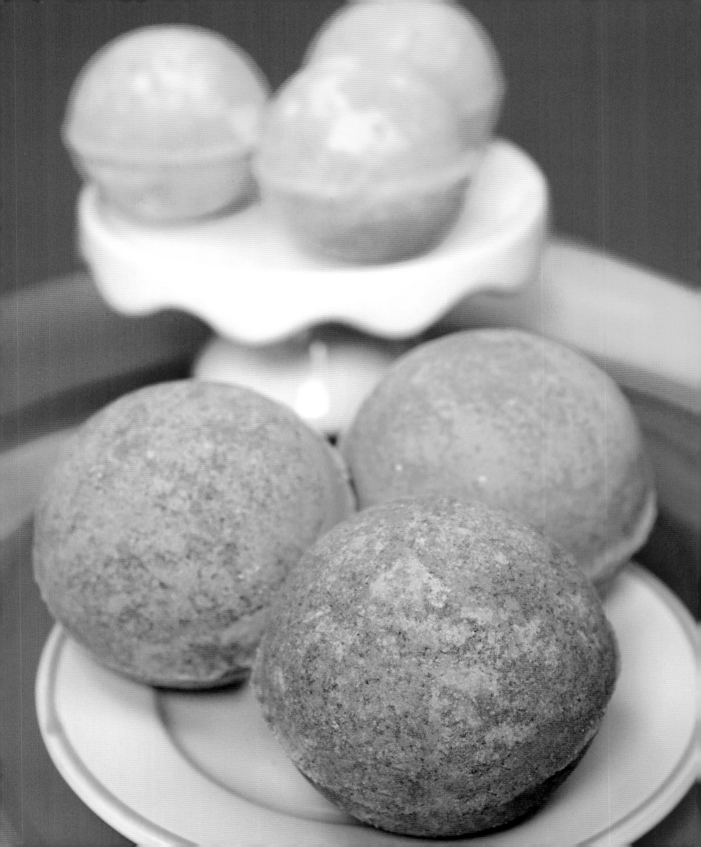

TIE-DYE
BATH BOMBS

Peace, love, and bath-time bliss are the ambitions of these multihued tie-dye bath bombs. Let happiness take over your heart as you unwind from the day and chase all your worries away with the fresh aroma of crisp white tea and ginger.

MAKES

10

BATH BOMBS

SUPPLIES

4 cups baking soda

½ cup cornstarch

3 tablespoons cream of tartar

1½ tablespoons sodium lauryl sulfoacetate (SLSA)

½ teaspoon each 4 mica colorants of choice

2 tablespoons sweet almond oil, divided

1 tablespoon polysorbate 80, divided

20 drops white tea and ginger fragrance oil

½ teaspoon water, divided

2 cups citric acid, divided

Witch hazel, scant amount as needed

Chopstick or similar item

2½″ round bath bomb mold

MIXING DIRECTIONS

1· In a large mixing bowl, thoroughly combine the baking soda, cornstarch, cream of tartar, and SLSA. Divide the mixture evenly into four medium bowls. Mix ½ teaspoon of mica colorant in the colors of your choice into each of the four bowls (a different color in each bowl).

2· In a small container, combine ½ tablespoon of the sweet almond oil, ¼ tablespoon of the polysorbate 80, 5 drops of the white tea and ginger fragrance oil, and ⅛ teaspoon of the water. Stirring constantly, slowly mix the liquids into the first bowl of dry ingredients until they are completely combined. Repeat for each of the different colored bowls.

3· Add ½ cup of the citric acid to each of the bowls and stir until it is fully incorporated into the mixture. If the mixture is not quite wet enough to mold, spritz two to three times with a spray bottle of witch hazel and mix well. Repeat as necessary.

MOLDING DIRECTIONS

4· Place small amounts of each color into both halves of the mold. Stir with a chopstick to mix the colors. Add more of each color and stir again until both sides of the mold are filled and mixed. Make sure to overfill the mold just a bit. Press the halves firmly together.

5· Carefully release the bath bomb from the mold and allow it to dry completely for 24–48 hours. Repeat to create the remaining bath bombs.

Hint· Tie-dye bath bombs are also a great way to use up any leftover bath bomb mixture at the end of your batch!

'80S SPLATTER-PAINTED
BATH BOMBS

Flash back to the time of boomboxes, neon, and big hair with these splatter-painted bath bombs! Don't be afraid to crank up the power ballads and settle into a bath-time experience that's sure to spark nostalgia as you drift away under the multicolored suds.

MAKES

BATH BOMBS

SUPPLIES

3 cups baking soda

2 tablespoons cream of tartar

2 tablespoons milk powder

1½ tablespoons sodium
  lauryl sulfoacetate (SLSA)

2 tablespoons grapeseed oil

1 tablespoon polysorbate 80

1 teaspoon coconut
  cream fragrance oil

1½ cups citric acid

Witch hazel, scant
  amount as needed

½ teaspoon isopropyl alcohol
  for each neon mica colorant

¼ teaspoon each of assorted
  neon mica colorants

2½" round bath bomb mold

MIXING DIRECTIONS

1 · In a large mixing bowl, thoroughly combine the baking soda, cream of tartar, milk powder, and SLSA.

2 · In a small container, mix together the grapeseed oil, polysorbate 80, and coconut cream fragrance oil. Stirring constantly, slowly mix the liquids into the dry ingredients until they are completely combined.

3 · Add the citric acid to the mixture and stir until it is fully incorporated. If the mixture is not quite wet enough to mold, spritz two to three times with a spray bottle of witch hazel and mix well. Repeat as necessary.

MOLDING DIRECTIONS

4 · Lightly overfill both halves of the mold with the mixture. Press the halves firmly together.

5 · Carefully release the bath bomb from the mold and allow it to dry completely for 24–48 hours. Repeat to create the remaining bath bombs.

6 · When the bath bombs are dry, mix ¼ teaspoon of each mica colorant with ½ teaspoon of the isopropyl alcohol and use a stiff paintbrush to splatter paint each bath bomb with a variety of neon colors.

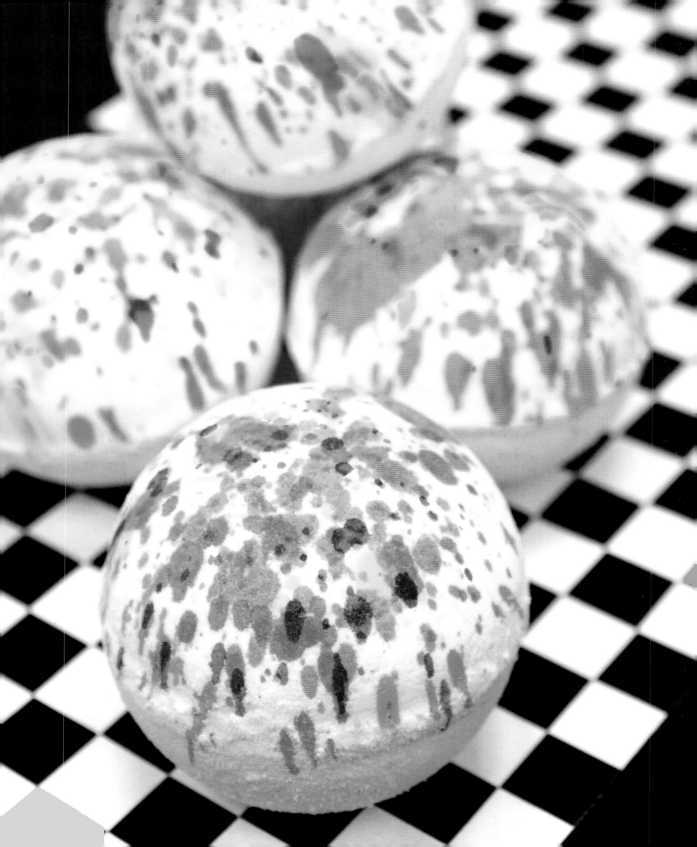

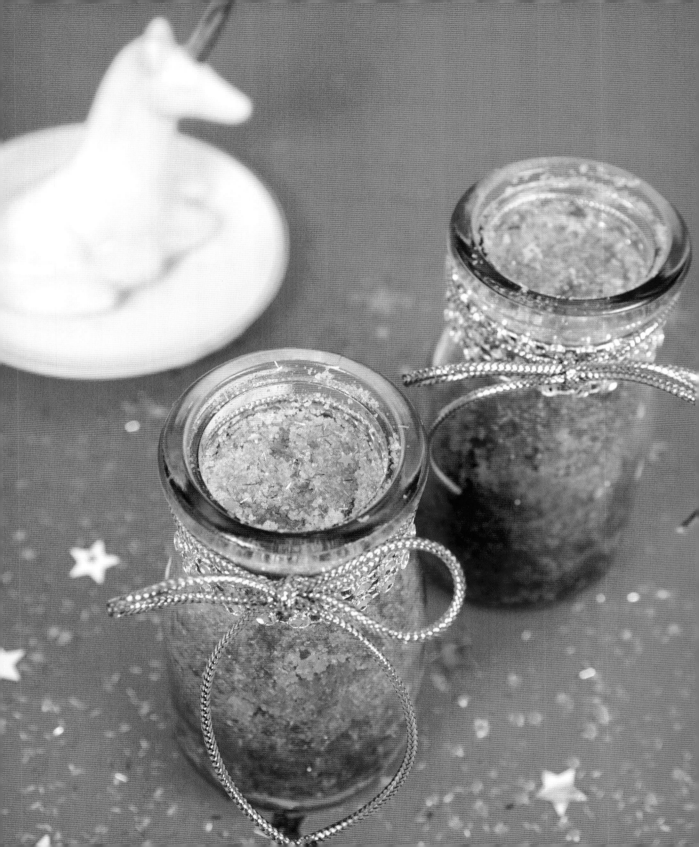

UNICORN
SHIMMER SCRUB

Let's be honest: you never really outgrow unicorns. This magical sugar scrub is a dream come true for all ages! Loaded with sparkle and shine, this fun body treatment is more than pretty; it also leaves your skin feeling silky smooth and smelling delicious.

MAKES

20 OUNCES

SUGAR SCRUB

SUPPLIES

2 cups granulated sugar, divided

⅛ teaspoon bright pink mica colorant

⅛ teaspoon purple mica colorant

⅛ teaspoon aqua mica colorant

1 teaspoon cosmetic grade glitter

1 cup fractionated coconut oil

20 drops bubblegum fragrance oil

Storage jars

Gold edible-glitter star sprinkles, optional

DIRECTIONS

1 · Divide the sugar into three small bowls. Stir just one color of mica colorant into each bowl. Add ⅓ teaspoon of the cosmetic glitter into each. Mix well until thoroughly combined.

2 · In another small bowl, mix together the fractionated coconut oil and bubblegum fragrance oil. Add ⅓ of the liquid mixture into each of the bowls of dry ingredients and stir until combined.

3 · Layer the different colors of sugar scrub into storage jars. Top with a light dusting of gold star sprinkles, if desired.

GEMSTONE
SOAPS

These opulent gemstone soaps sparkle and shine with posh splendor. Let the lavish and luxurious fragrances of champagne and raspberries sweep you away to palatial fantasies every time you wash up!

MAKES

10

SOAPS

SUPPLIES

1 pound crystal clear soap base

Microwave-safe measuring cup

6 drops each soap colorant
  in red, gold, green,
  blue, and purple

25 drops champagne
  fragrance oil

25 drops raspberry fragrance oil

Isopropyl alcohol, in
  a spray bottle

Silicone gemstone soap mold

DIRECTIONS

1· Slice the crystal clear soap base into small cubes and divide into five equal piles. Place the first batch of soap cubes into a microwave-safe measuring cup. Melt in the microwave in 30-second increments, stirring well after each session to ensure that the soap is completely melted.

2· Carefully stir in 6 drops of red soap colorant, 5 drops of the champagne fragrance oil, and 5 drops of the raspberry fragrance oil. Pour the melted soap into two wells of the mold and spritz with isopropyl alcohol to remove any air bubbles. Allow to cool for 20 minutes. Repeat the process for each different color of soap.

3· Allow the soaps to sit undisturbed until completely firm (approximately 30–90 minutes depending on temperature and humidity) before unmolding.

SPLASHES

OF FUN

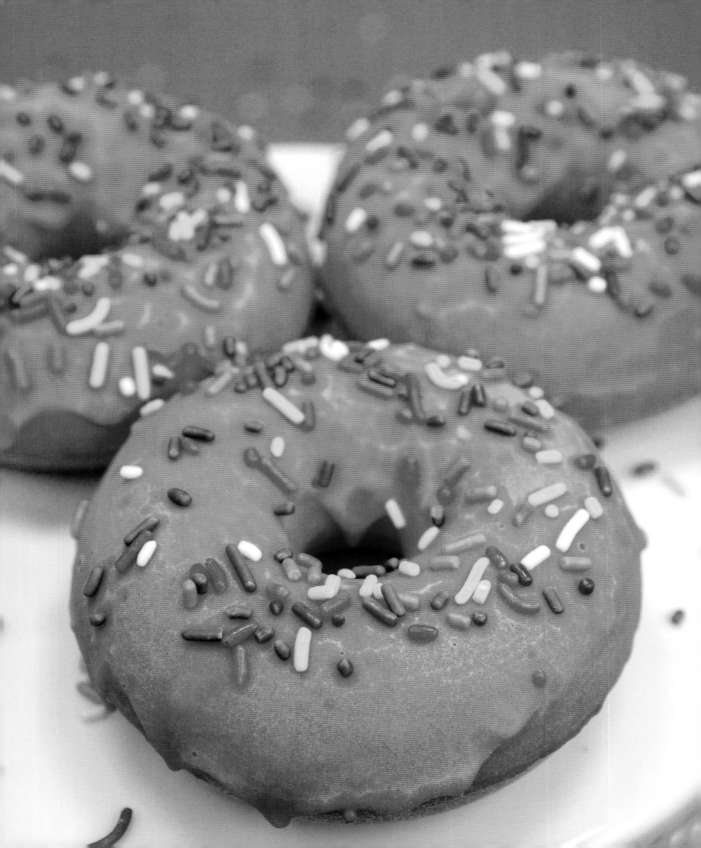

DONUT
BATH BOMBS

Who knew donuts could work wonders for your skin? Topped with a thick layer of sumptuous cocoa butter icing, these bath bombs deliver a moisturizing and skin-smoothing spa treatment in your own bathtub. And the scent is straight from the bakery!

MAKES

5

BATH BOMBS

SUPPLIES

4 cups baking soda, divided

2 tablespoons cream of tartar

2½ tablespoons sodium lauryl sulfoacetate (SLSA)

½ teaspoon gold mica colorant

2 tablespoons sweet almond oil

1 tablespoon polysorbate 80

1 teaspoon coffee cake fragrance oil

½ teaspoon water

1½ cups citric acid

Witch hazel, scant amount as needed

3-piece donut bath bomb mold

1 cup cocoa butter, melted

2 drops pink candy color

Sprinkles

MIXING DIRECTIONS

1 · In a large mixing bowl, thoroughly combine 3 cups of the baking soda, the cream of tartar, SLSA, and gold mica.

2 · In a small container, stir together the sweet almond oil, polysorbate 80, coffee cake fragrance oil, and water. Stirring constantly, slowly add the liquids into the dry ingredients until they are completely combined.

3 · Add the citric acid to the mixture and stir until it is fully incorporated. If the mixture is not quite wet enough to mold, spritz two to three times with a spray bottle of witch hazel and mix well. Repeat as necessary.

MOLDING DIRECTIONS

4 · Place the bottom half of the mold inside the molding ring. Loosely pack the bath bomb mixture inside the mold and continue to fill the remainder of the mold, overfilling just slightly. Press the top half of the mold firmly into the ring. Flip the mold over and press again from the opposite side. Slide the ring off the mold and carefully unmold the bath bomb. Allow to dry completely for 24–48 hours. Repeat to create the remaining bath bombs.

5 · When the bath bombs are dry, melt the cocoa butter and slowly add up to 1 cup of baking soda until you reach an icing-like consistency. Add the pink candy color. Pour the cocoa butter icing into a shallow bowl, then dip the top of each donut bath bomb in the icing. Add sprinkles while the icing is still wet. Allow to dry and harden for at least 3 hours.

STRAWBERRY MILKSHAKE
BATH BOMBS

Milk powder, coconut oil, and colloidal oats make these bath bombs a splendid treat for your skin! Fill your tub with pink-tinted fizz and take it easy under a luxurious layer of frothy bubbles and the sweet, indulgent aroma!

MAKES

BATH BOMBS

SUPPLIES

4 cups baking soda, divided

2 tablespoons cream of tartar

2½ tablespoons milk powder

3 tablespoons colloidal oats

1 teaspoon pink mica colorant

2 tablespoons coconut
  oil, melted

1 tablespoon polysorbate 80

1 teaspoon strawberry
  fragrance oil

¼ teaspoon vanilla fragrance oil

½ teaspoon water

1½ cups citric acid

Witch hazel, scant
  amount as needed

¼ cup cocamidopropyl betaine

Sprinkles

6 4-ounce paper cups

Piping bag and tip

Paper straws, cut into 2″ pieces

Mixer

Mixing Directions

1 · In a large mixing bowl, thoroughly combine 3 cups of the baking soda with the cream of tartar, milk powder, colloidal oats, and pink mica.

2 · In a small container, stir together the melted coconut oil, polysorbate 80, strawberry fragrance oil, vanilla fragrance oil, and water. Stirring constantly, slowly add the liquids into the dry ingredients until they are completely combined.

3 · Add the citric acid to the mixture and stir until it is fully incorporated. If the mixture is not quite wet enough to mold, spritz two to three times with a spray bottle of witch hazel and mix well. Repeat as necessary.

MOLDING DIRECTIONS

4 · Press the bath bomb mixture firmly into the paper cups using your thumb and the palm of your hand to apply pressure. Fill the cups to the top until they are packed completely full.

5 · Carefully release the bath bombs from the cups and allow them to dry completely for 24–48 hours. Alternately, you can allow the bath bombs to dry overnight in the cups and then unmold.

6 · Use a mixer to make bubble icing by whipping together the cocamidopropyl betaine and 1 cup of the baking soda. Depending on humidity and temperature, you may need to add more baking soda or cocamidopropyl betaine until your bubble icing reaches a pipeable consistency. Transfer the mixture to a piping bag and top each milkshake bath bomb with a swirl of icing. Add sprinkles while the icing is still wet and insert a paper straw. Allow to dry and harden for at least 24 hours.

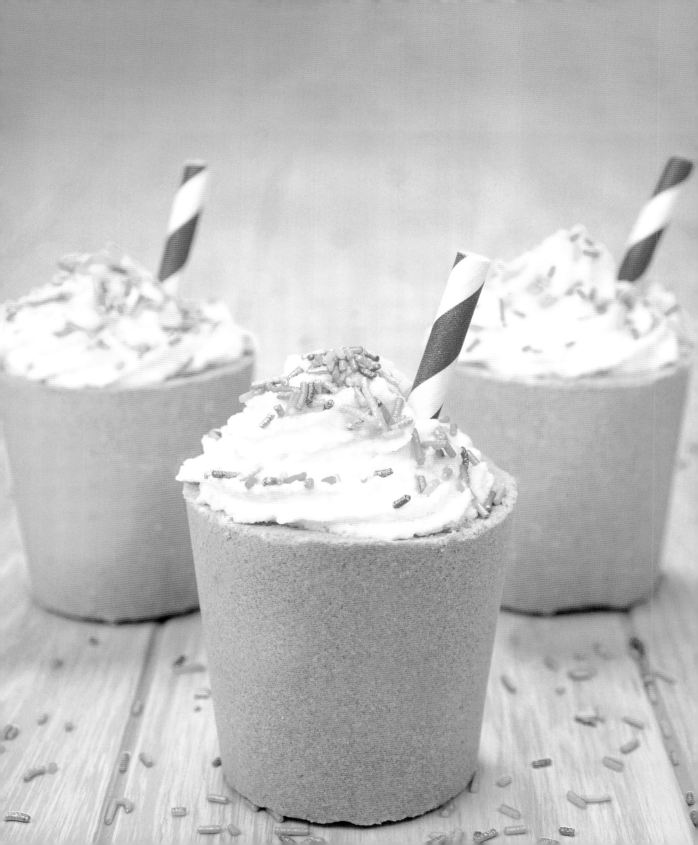

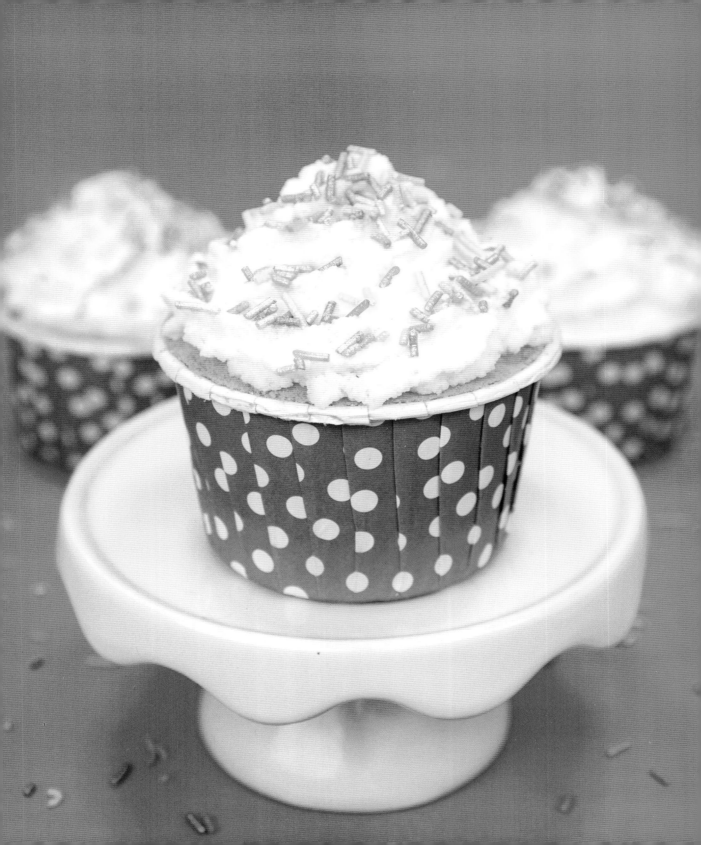

CUPCAKE
BATH BOMBS

Celebrate every day in birthday style with these adorable bath bombs! Topped with a generous swirl of bubble frosting, these cupcakes deliver lavish loads of silky bubbles layered on top of pretty pink fizz for a decadent bath-time experience.

MAKES

BATH BOMBS

SUPPLIES

4 cups baking soda, divided

1 cup cornstarch

1 cup Epsom salt, finely ground

2 tablespoons white kaolin clay

2½ tablespoons sodium lauryl sulfoacetate (SLSA)

1 teaspoon bright pink mica colorant

2½ tablespoons sweet almond oil

1 tablespoon polysorbate 80

1 teaspoon cupcake fragrance oil

1½ cups citric acid

Witch hazel, scant amount as needed

¼ cup cocamidopropyl betaine

Sprinkles

Paper treat cups

Piping bag and tip

Mixer

MIXING DIRECTIONS

1 · In a large mixing bowl, thoroughly combine 3 cups of the baking soda with the cornstarch, Epsom salt, kaolin clay, SLSA, and bright pink mica.

2 · In a small container, stir together the sweet almond oil, polysorbate 80, and cupcake fragrance oil. Stirring constantly, slowly add the liquids into the dry ingredients until they are completely combined.

3 · Add the citric acid to the mixture and stir until it is fully incorporated. If the mixture is not quite wet enough to mold, spritz two to three times with a spray bottle of witch hazel and mix well. Repeat as necessary.

MOLDING DIRECTIONS

4 · Press the bath bomb mixture firmly into the paper cups using your thumb and the palm of your hand to apply pressure. Fill the cups to the top until they are packed completely full.

5 · Carefully release the bath bombs from the cups and allow them to dry completely for 24–48 hours. Alternately, you can allow the bath bombs to dry overnight in the cups and then unmold.

6 · Use a mixer to make bubble icing by whipping together cocamido-propyl betaine and 1 cup of the baking soda. Depending on humidity and temperature, you may need to add more baking soda or cocamido-propyl betaine until your bubble icing reaches a pipeable consistency. Transfer the mixture to a piping bag and top each cupcake bath bomb with a swirl of icing. Add sprinkles while the icing is still wet. Allow to dry and harden for at least 24 hours.

COTTON CANDY
BATH BOMBS

How sweet it is to bring this nostalgic candy-scented aroma to bath time! Relax without a care in the world as you soak in a tub full of soft foam that will make you feel as though you're floating in a cloud of cotton candy itself.

MAKES

BATH BOMBS

SUPPLIES

3 cups baking soda

1 cup Epsom salt, finely ground

2½ tablespoons cream of tartar

3 tablespoons sodium lauryl sulfoacetate (SLSA)

1 teaspoon bright blue mica colorant

1 teaspoon pink mica colorant

2 tablespoons fractionated coconut oil, divided

1 tablespoon polysorbate 80, divided

½ teaspoon water, divided

1 teaspoon cotton candy fragrance oil, divided

1½ cups citric acid, divided

Witch hazel, scant amount as needed

2½" round bath bomb mold

MIXING DIRECTIONS

1 · In a large mixing bowl, thoroughly combine the baking soda, Epsom salt, cream of tartar, and SLSA. Divide the mixture evenly into two medium bowls. Mix the blue mica into one bowl and the pink mica into the second bowl.

2 · In a small container, combine 1 tablespoon of the fractionated coconut oil, ½ tablespoon of the polysorbate 80, ¼ teaspoon of the water, and ½ teaspoon of the cotton candy fragrance oil. Stirring constantly, slowly mix the liquids into the blue dry ingredients until they are completely combined. Repeat for the pink mixture.

3 · Add ¾ cup of the citric acid to each of the bowls and stir until it is fully incorporated into the mixture. If the mixture is not quite wet enough to mold, spritz two to three times with a spray bottle of witch hazel and mix well. Repeat as necessary.

MOLDING DIRECTIONS

4 · Fill half of the mold with the blue bath bomb mixture and the other half with pink. Make sure to overfill the mold just a bit. Press the halves firmly together.

5 · Carefully release the bath bomb from the mold and allow it to dry completely for 24–48 hours. Repeat to create the remaining bath bombs.

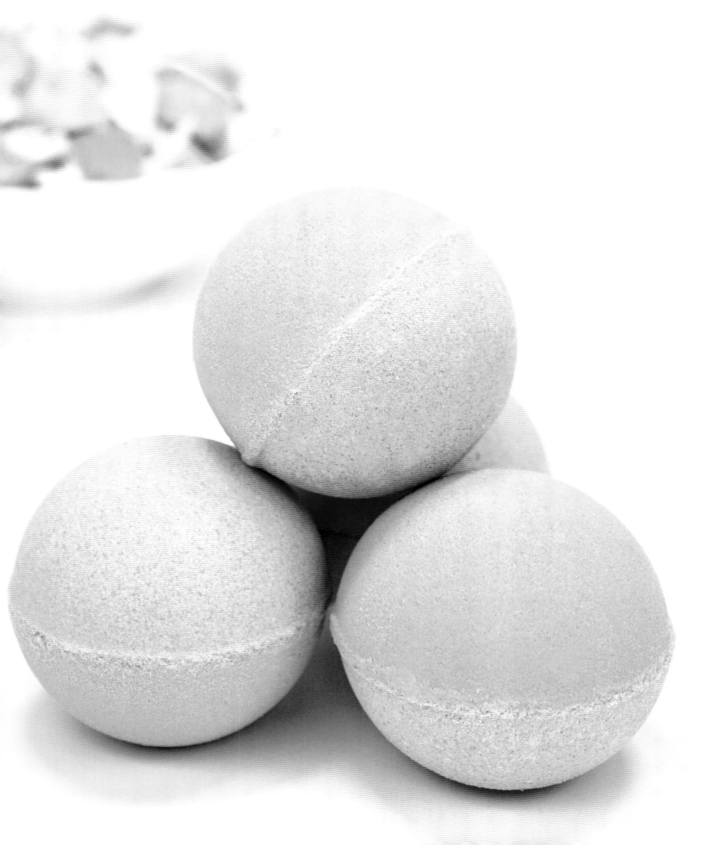

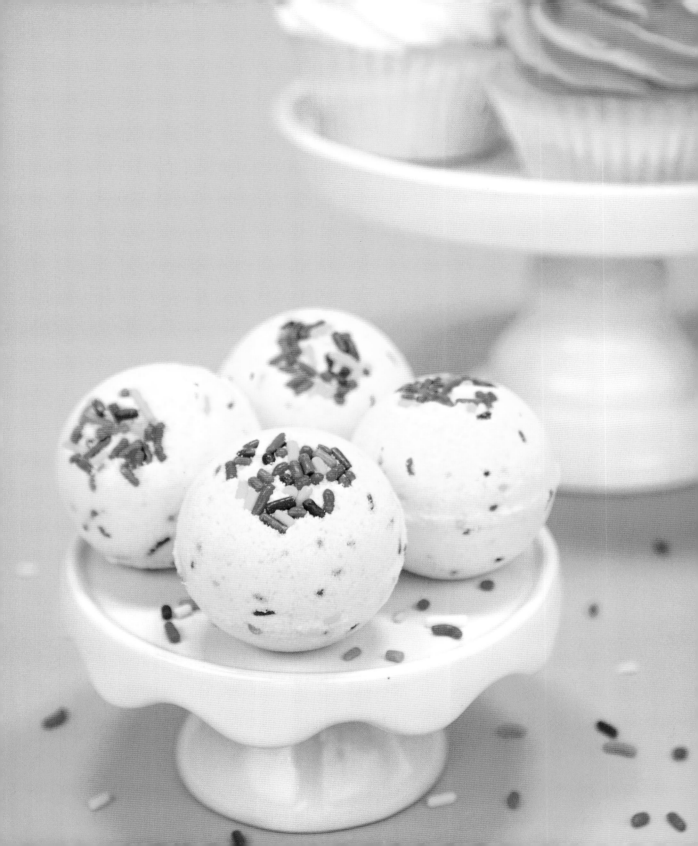

BIRTHDAY CAKE
BATH BOMBS

Birthday cake should be enjoyed every day, don't you think? These charming birthday cake bath bombs are loaded with sweet sprinkles and a bakery-fresh aroma that will make you forget all your troubles. Coconut oil nourishes dry skin and smells incredible.

MAKES

BATH BOMBS

SUPPLIES

1½ cups baking soda

1 tablespoon cream of tartar

1 tablespoon white kaolin clay

⅓ cup cornstarch

1½ tablespoons sodium lauryl sulfoacetate (SLSA)

⅛ teaspoon yellow mica colorant

1½ tablespoons coconut oil, melted

½ tablespoon polysorbate 80

½ teaspoon cupcake fragrance oil

¼ teaspoon buttercream fragrance oil

¾ cups citric acid

Sprinkles

Witch hazel, scant amount as needed

2″ round bath bomb mold

MIXING DIRECTIONS

1 · In a large mixing bowl, thoroughly combine the baking soda, cream of tartar, kaolin clay, cornstarch, SLSA, and yellow mica.

2 · In a small container, mix together the melted coconut oil, polysorbate 80, cupcake fragrance oil, and buttercream fragrance oil. Stirring constantly, slowly mix the liquids into the dry ingredients until they are completely combined.

3 · Add the citric acid to the mixture and stir until it is fully incorporated. Mix in 2 tablespoons of the sprinkles. If the mixture is not quite wet enough to mold, spritz two to three times with a spray bottle of witch hazel and mix well. Repeat as necessary.

MOLDING DIRECTIONS

4 · Start by adding a large pinch of sprinkles to the bottom of one half of the mold. Lightly pack both halves of the mold, making sure to slightly overfill each half. Press the halves firmly together.

5 · Carefully release the bath bomb from the mold and allow it to dry completely for 24–48 hours. Repeat to create the remaining bath bombs.

JUICE BOX
BATH BOMBS

Juice box bath bombs are a darling way to make bath-time fun! The crisp aroma of fresh apples will delight your senses as you unwind in a blissful bath of bright green fizz and frothy bubbles.

MAKES

BATH BOMBS

SUPPLIES

3 cups baking soda

2 tablespoons cream of tartar

2 tablespoons sodium lauryl sulfoacetate (SLSA)

1 teaspoon green mica colorant

2 tablespoons sweet almond oil

1 tablespoon polysorbate 80

1 teaspoon apple fragrance oil

½ teaspoon water

1½ cups citric acid

Witch hazel, scant amount as needed

Paper straws

3-piece rectangle bath bomb mold

MIXING DIRECTIONS

1 · In a large mixing bowl, thoroughly combine the baking soda, cream of tartar, SLSA, and green mica.

2 · In a small container, stir together the sweet almond oil, polysorbate 80, apple fragrance oil, and water. Stirring constantly, slowly add the liquids into the dry ingredients until they are completely combined.

3 · Add the citric acid to the mixture and stir until it is fully incorporated. If the mixture is not quite wet enough to mold, spritz two to three times with a spray bottle of witch hazel and mix well. Repeat as necessary.

MOLDING DIRECTIONS

4 · Place the bottom half of the mold inside the molding ring. Loosely pack the bath bomb mixture inside the mold and continue to fill the remainder of the mold, overfilling just slightly. Press the top half of the mold firmly into the ring. Flip the mold over and press again from the opposite side. Slide the ring off the mold and carefully unmold the bath bomb. Insert a paper straw into the top and allow to dry completely for 24–48 hours. Repeat to create the remaining bath bombs.

5 · When the bath bombs are dry, add a juice box label. You can download label designs at happinessishomemade.com/juice-box-labels.

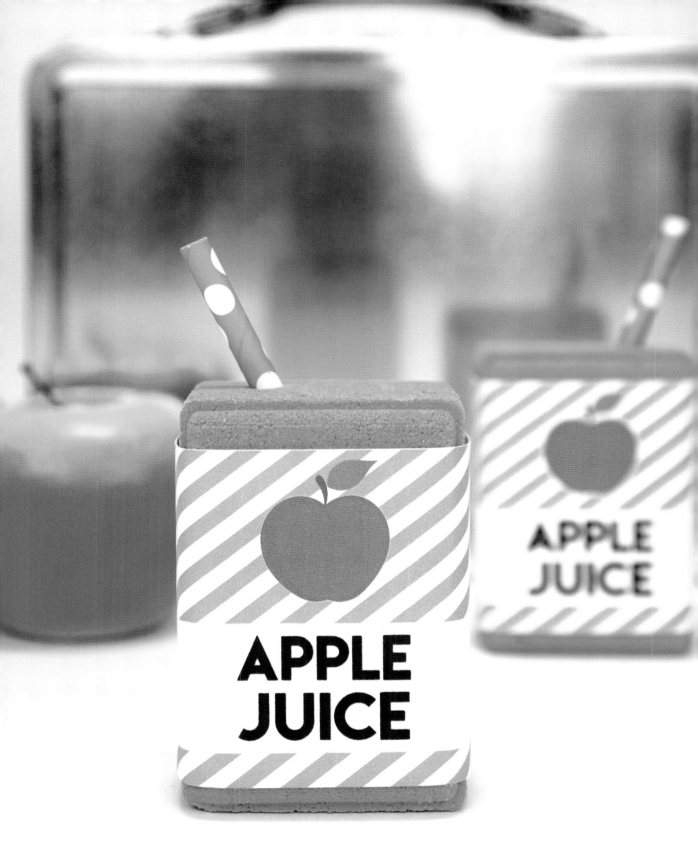

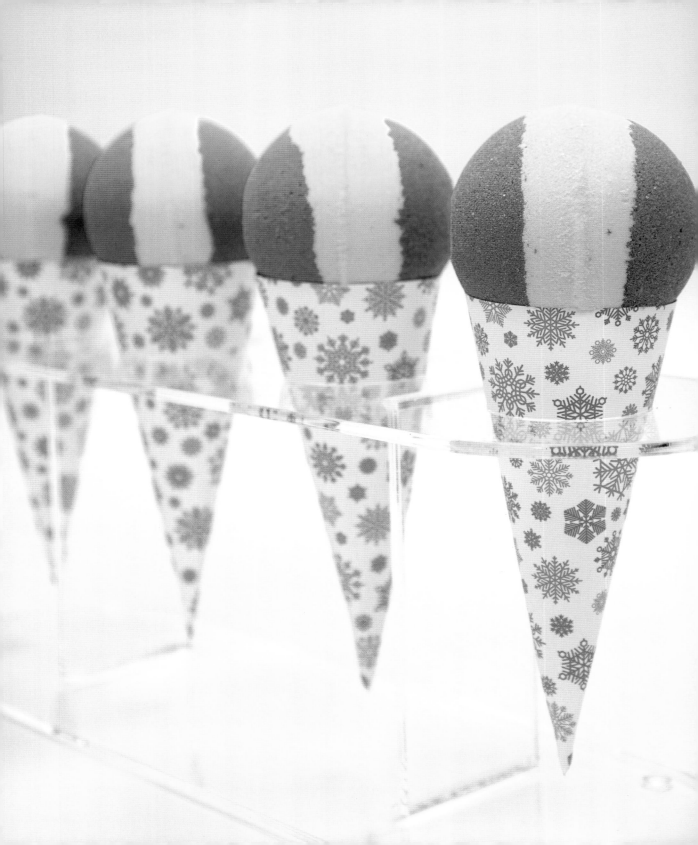

SNOW CONE
BATH BOMBS

Snow cones are a refreshing summer treat, and these snow cone bath bombs are just as refreshing in your tub! Let the fruity fragrances blast away your troubles as you soak beneath the sweet-scented fizz!

MAKES

15

BATH BOMBS

SUPPLIES

5 cups baking soda

1 cup cornstarch

1 cup Epsom salt

3 tablespoons cream of tartar

3 tablespoons sodium lauryl sulfoacetate (SLSA)

1 teaspoon red mica colorant

1 teaspoon yellow mica colorant

1 teaspoon blue mica colorant

3 tablespoons sweet almond oil, divided

3 tablespoons polysorbate 80, divided

1 teaspoon strawberry fragrance oil

1 teaspoon banana fragrance oil

1 teaspoon blueberry fragrance oil

3 cups citric acid, divided

Witch hazel, scant amount as needed

2½" round bath bomb mold

MIXING DIRECTIONS

1 · In a large mixing bowl, thoroughly combine the baking soda, cornstarch, Epsom salt, cream of tartar, and SLSA. Divide the mixture evenly into three medium bowls. Mix the red mica into one bowl, the yellow into the second bowl, and the blue into the third.

2 · In a small container, combine 1 tablespoon of the sweet almond oil, 1 tablespoon of the polysorbate 80, and the strawberry fragrance oil. Stirring constantly, slowly mix the liquids into the red dry ingredients.

3 · In another small container, combine 1 tablespoon of the sweet almond oil, 1 tablespoon of the polysorbate 80, and the banana fragrance oil. Stirring constantly, slowly mix the liquids into the yellow dry ingredients.

4 · In a third small container, combine the remaining sweet almond oil and polysorbate 80 with the blueberry fragrance oil. Stirring constantly, slowly mix the liquids into the blue dry ingredients.

5 · Stir 1 cup of the citric acid into each of the bowls. If the mixture is not quite wet enough to mold, spritz two to three times with a spray bottle of witch hazel and mix well. Repeat as necessary.

MOLDING DIRECTIONS

6 · Layer the mixtures into both halves of the mold in a striped pattern. Make sure to overfill the mold just a bit. Press the halves firmly together.

7 · Carefully release the bath bomb from the mold and allow it to dry completely for 24–48 hours. Repeat to create the remaining bath bombs.

8 · Package the bath bombs with printable cones from happinessishomemade.net/snow-cone-printables.

MONSTER
BATH BOMBS

*M*ake bath time extra fun with these bath bombs! The charming monster family will bring smiles to both the young and young at heart. This recipe makes one color of monster; repeat the process for a rainbow of spooky friends.

MAKES

7

BATH BOMBS

SUPPLIES

1½ cups baking soda

2 tablespoons cream of tartar

1½ tablespoons sodium lauryl sulfoacetate (SLSA)

½ teaspoon teal mica colorant

1½ tablespoons fractionated coconut oil

½ tablespoon polysorbate 80

1 teaspoon key lime fragrance oil

¾ cups citric acid

Witch hazel, scant amount as needed

2″ round bath bomb mold

Candy eyes

MIXING DIRECTIONS

1 · In a large mixing bowl, thoroughly combine the baking soda, cream of tartar, SLSA, and teal mica.

2 · In a small container, mix together the fractionated coconut oil, polysorbate 80, and key lime fragrance oil. Stirring constantly, slowly mix the liquids into the dry ingredients until they are completely combined.

3 · Add the citric acid to the mixture and stir until it is fully incorporated. If the mixture is not quite wet enough to mold, spritz two to three times with a spray bottle of witch hazel and mix well. Repeat as necessary.

MOLDING DIRECTIONS

4 · Start by adding a candy eye or two to the side of one half of the mold. Lightly pack both halves of the mold, making sure to slightly overfill each half. Press the halves firmly together.

5 · Carefully release the bath bomb from the mold and allow it to dry completely for 24–48 hours. Repeat to create the remaining bath bombs.

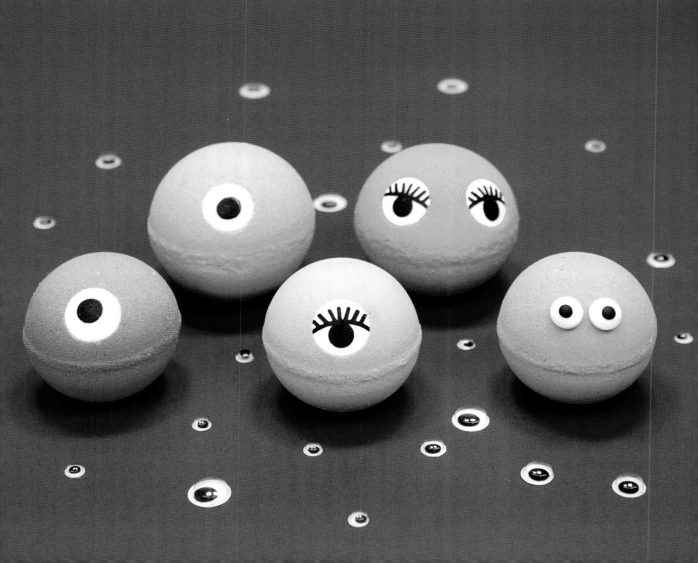

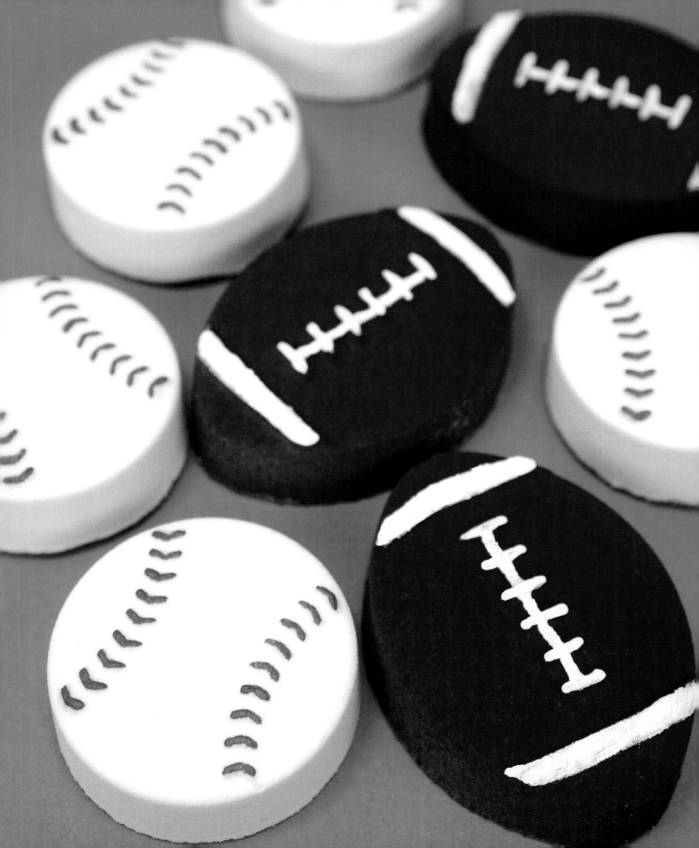

SPORTS BALL
BATH BOMBS

These bath bombs are the perfect post-game celebration! Epsom salt helps relax achy muscles and loosen stiff joints after a tough game or workout. Feel free to swap out the root beer and experiment with a stronger scent like leather or stout.

MAKES

10

BATH BOMBS

SUPPLIES

2 cups baking soda

1 cup Epsom salt, finely ground

2 tablespoons cream of tartar

1 tablespoon white kaolin clay

1½ tablespoons sodium lauryl sulfoacetate (SLSA)

2 tablespoons sweet almond oil

½ tablespoon polysorbate 80

1 teaspoon root beer fragrance oil

Dash of French vanilla fragrance oil

1 cup citric acid

Witch hazel, scant amount as needed

Hard plastic baseball and football molds

2 teaspoons isopropyl alcohol, divided

½ teaspoon brown mica colorant

¼ teaspoon white mica colorant

¼ teaspoon red mica colorant

MIXING DIRECTIONS

1 · In a large mixing bowl, thoroughly combine the baking soda, Epsom salt, cream of tartar, kaolin clay, and SLSA.

2 · In a small container, mix together the sweet almond oil, polysorbate 80, root beer fragrance oil, and French vanilla fragrance oil. Stirring constantly, slowly mix the liquids into the dry ingredients until they are completely combined.

3 · Add the citric acid to the mixture and stir until it is fully incorporated. If the mixture is not quite wet enough to mold, spritz two to three times with a spray bottle of witch hazel and mix well. Repeat as necessary.

MOLDING DIRECTIONS

4 · Press the bath bomb mixture firmly into the molds using your thumb and the palm of your hand to apply pressure. Fill the molds to the top until they are packed completely full.

5 · Carefully release the bath bombs from the mold and allow them to dry completely for 24–48 hours.

6 · When the bath bombs are dry, mix 1 teaspoon of the isopropyl alcohol with the brown mica in a misting spray bottle. Spray the footballs with the brown mica paint. Mix the white mica with ½ teaspoon of the isopropyl alcohol and use a paintbrush to apply the white details to the footballs. Mix the red mica with ½ teaspoon of the isopropyl alcohol and use a paintbrush to apply the red lacing details to the baseballs.

PAW PRINT
BATH BOMBS

Calling all animal lovers! These "paw-some" bath bombs are a real treat for your skin. Activated charcoal gently exfoliates and deep cleans pores while the exotic kukui nut oil delivers advanced antiaging properties and deep hydration.

MAKES

BATH BOMBS

SUPPLIES

3 cups baking soda

2½ tablespoons cream of tartar

1 tablespoon arrowroot powder

2 tablespoons sodium lauryl sulfoacetate (SLSA)

1 tablespoon activated charcoal powder

2 tablespoons kukui nut oil, divided

1 tablespoon polysorbate 80, divided

½ teaspoon water, divided

1 teaspoon rose garden fragrance oil, divided

1½ cups citric acid, divided

Witch hazel, scant amount as needed

Hard plastic paw print mold

¼ teaspoon pink pearl mica

½ teaspoon isopropyl alcohol

MIXING DIRECTIONS

1 · In a large mixing bowl, thoroughly combine the baking soda, cream of tartar, arrowroot powder, and SLSA. Divide the mixture evenly into two medium bowls. Mix the activated charcoal powder into one bowl and leave the second bowl uncolored.

2 · In a small container, combine 1 tablespoon of the kukui nut oil, ½ tablespoon of the polysorbate 80, ¼ teaspoon of the water, and ½ teaspoon of the rose garden fragrance oil. Stirring constantly, slowly mix the liquids into the black dry ingredients until they are completely combined. Repeat for the white mixture.

3 · Add ¾ cup of the citric acid to each of the bowls and stir until it is fully incorporated into the mixture. If the mixture is not quite wet enough to mold, spritz two to three times with a spray bottle of witch hazel and mix well. Repeat as necessary.

MOLDING DIRECTIONS

4 · Press the bath bomb mixture firmly into the mold using your thumb and the palm of your hand to apply pressure. Fill the mold to the top until it is packed completely full.

5 · Carefully release the bath bomb from the mold and allow it to dry completely for 24–48 hours. Repeat to create the remaining bath bombs.

6 · When the bath bombs are dry, mix the pink pearl mica with the isopropyl alcohol and use a paintbrush to add details to the paw prints. ***Note*** • *For human use only; not for use on pets.*

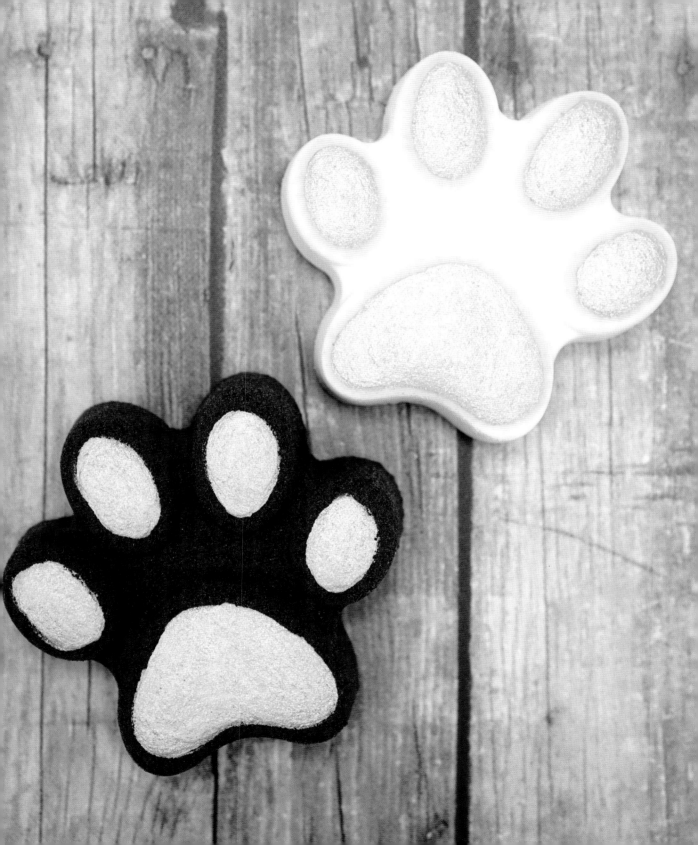

BABY-FRIENDLY
BATH BOMBS

Young children love the fizzing action of bath bombs, and these gentle bath bombs are specially formulated to be safe even for babies. The fizzy pink water will delight their senses, and the jojoba oil delivers soothing hydration for ultrasensitive skin.

MAKES

5

BATH BOMBS

SUPPLIES

3 cups baking soda

1 cup cornstarch

2 tablespoons cream of tartar

¼ teaspoon pink mica colorant

2½ tablespoons jojoba oil

1 tablespoon tear-free
baby shampoo

1½ cups citric acid

Witch hazel, scant
amount as needed

3″ round bath bomb mold

MIXING DIRECTIONS

1 • In a large mixing bowl, thoroughly combine the baking soda, cornstarch, cream of tartar, and pink mica.

2 • In a small container, mix together the jojoba oil and baby shampoo. Stirring constantly, slowly mix the liquids into the dry ingredients until they are completely combined.

3 • Add the citric acid to the mixture and stir until it is fully incorporated. If the mixture is not quite wet enough to mold, spritz two to three times with a spray bottle of witch hazel and mix well. Repeat as necessary.

MOLDING DIRECTIONS

4 • Lightly overfill both halves of the mold with the mixture. Press the halves firmly together.

5 • Carefully release the bath bomb from the mold and allow it to dry completely for 24–48 hours. Repeat to create the remaining bath bombs.

DONUT
SOAPS

Just a few simple ingredients can transform into an amazing treat! Pamper yourself with lush and hydrating goat's milk soap and the comforting scent of fresh baked goods. You won't believe it took you so long to discover this soap.

MAKES

SOAPS

SUPPLIES

Silicone donut mold

Sprinkles

1½ pounds goat's milk soap base

Microwave-safe measuring cup

2 drops wine soap colorant

1 teaspoon cupcake fragrance oil, divided

Isopropyl alcohol, in a spray bottle

6 drops gold soap colorant

DIRECTIONS

1 · Fill the bottom of the donut mold with a thin layer of sprinkles.

2 · Slice the goat's milk soap base into small cubes and place ½ pound of the cubes into a microwave-safe measuring cup. Melt in the microwave in 30-second increments, stirring well after each session to ensure that the soap is completely melted.

3 · Carefully stir in the wine soap colorant and ½ teaspoon cupcake fragrance oil. Pour the melted soap into the mold and spritz with isopropyl alcohol to remove any air bubbles. Allow to cool for 15–20 minutes.

4 · Melt the remaining cubes of soap base in the microwave, and carefully stir in the gold soap colorant and the remaining ½ teaspoon of cupcake fragrance oil. Spritz the pink layer of soap with isopropyl alcohol (to help the layers stick together), pour the gold soap into the molds, and spritz with isopropyl alcohol to remove any air bubbles.

5 · Allow the soaps to sit undisturbed until completely firm (approximately 60–90 minutes depending on temperature and humidity) before unmolding.

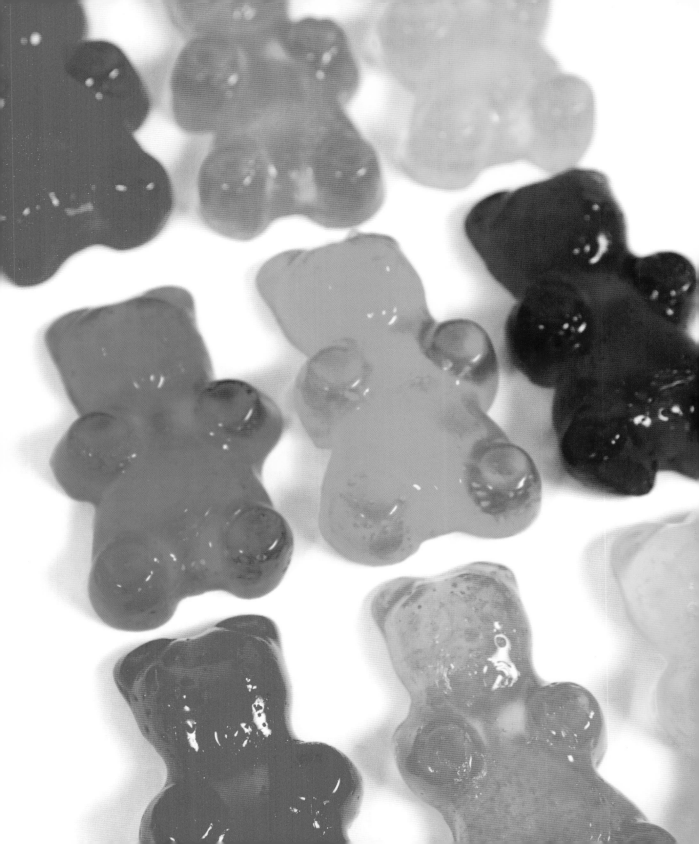

GUMMY BEAR
SHOWER JELLIES

Sort of like a combo of soap and gelatin, jellies bring a playful touch to your shower. Mix and match your favorite color and fruity fragrance combinations or try something silly like pairing a red gummy bear with a lemon scent.

MAKES

18

SHOWER JELLIES

SUPPLIES

1 pound clear jelly soap base

Microwave-safe measuring cup

6 drops each soap colorant in red, orange, yellow, green, blue, and purple

10 drops each 6 assorted fruit-scented fragrance oils

Isopropyl alcohol, in a spray bottle

Large silicone gummy bear mold

DIRECTIONS

1 · Slice the jelly soap base into small cubes and divide into six equal piles. Place the first batch of soap cubes into a microwave-safe measuring cup. Melt in the microwave in 30-second increments, stirring well after each session to ensure that the soap is completely melted.

2 · Carefully stir in 6 drops of the red soap colorant and 10 drops of a fruit fragrance oil (cherry or strawberry would work great with the red color). Pour the melted soap into three wells of the mold and spritz with isopropyl alcohol to remove any air bubbles. Allow the soaps to sit undisturbed until completely firm (approximately 60–90 minutes depending on temperature and humidity) before unmolding.

3 · Repeat the process for each different color of soap, using a fruit fragrance oil to correspond to the color of the shower jelly.

RAINBOW
BATH CRAYONS

Let your inner Picasso loose in the tub and create a masterpiece in your bathroom with these bold-colored bath crayons! Soap-based bath crayons turn bath time into playtime and then wash away easily from skin and the tub, leaving everything squeaky clean!

MAKES

18

CRAYONS

SUPPLIES

1 pound shea butter soap base

Microwave-safe measuring cup

20 drops each food coloring in red, orange, yellow, green, blue, and purple

Isopropyl alcohol, in a spray bottle

2 silicone ice stick molds

DIRECTIONS

1 · Slice the shea butter soap base into small cubes and divide into six equal piles. Place the first batch of soap cubes into a microwave-safe measuring cup. Melt in the microwave in 30-second increments, stirring well after each session to ensure that the soap is completely melted.

2 · Carefully stir in the red food coloring. Pour the melted soap into three wells of the mold and spritz with isopropyl alcohol to remove any air bubbles. Allow the bath crayons to sit undisturbed until completely firm (approximately 30–90 minutes depending on temperature and humidity) before unmolding.

3 · Repeat the process for each different color of bath crayon.

CHAPTER SIX

HEALING

BATH

SWEET DREAMS
BATH BOMBS

You may already use a warm bath as a means to help bring on sleep. These bath bombs add extra relaxation to your tub with violet-colored water and creamy bath foam. The shea butter will nourish your skin as the essential oil blend carries you away to bedtime.

MAKES

BATH BOMBS

SUPPLIES

4 cups baking soda

½ cup cornstarch

2 tablespoons cream of tartar

2 tablespoons white kaolin clay

2 tablespoons sodium lauryl sulfoacetate (SLSA)

½ teaspoon purple mica colorant

½ teaspoon blue mica colorant

½ teaspoon green mica colorant

½ teaspoon teal mica colorant

2 tablespoons coconut oil, melted and divided

2 tablespoons shea butter, melted and divided

1 tablespoon polysorbate 80, divided

20 drops lavender essential oil

20 drops Roman chamomile essential oil

12 drops bergamot essential oil

12 drops ylang-ylang essential oil

2 cups citric acid, divided

Witch hazel, scant amount as needed

2½″ round bath bomb molds

Gold edible-glitter star sprinkles

MIXING DIRECTIONS

1 · In a large mixing bowl, thoroughly combine the baking soda, cornstarch, cream of tartar, kaolin clay, and SLSA. Divide the mixture evenly into four medium bowls. Mix the purple mica into one bowl, the blue into the second bowl, the green into the third bowl, and the teal into the fourth bowl.

2 · In a small container, combine ½ tablespoon of the melted coconut oil, ½ tablespoon of the melted shea butter, ¼ tablespoon of the polysorbate 80, 5 drops of the lavender essential oil, 5 drops of the Roman chamomile essential oil, 3 drops of the bergamot essential oil, and 3 drops of the ylang-ylang essential oil. Stirring constantly, slowly mix the liquids into the purple dry ingredients until they are completely combined. Repeat this step for each of the different colored bowls.

$3 \cdot$ Add ½ cup of the citric acid to each of the bowls and stir until it is fully incorporated into the mixture. If the mixture is not quite wet enough to mold, spritz two to three times with a spray bottle of witch hazel and mix well. Repeat as necessary.

MOLDING DIRECTIONS

$4 \cdot$ Start by adding a pinch of gold star sprinkles to the bottom of one half of the mold. Lightly pack both halves of the mold in a striped pattern, making sure to slightly overfill each half. Press the halves firmly together.

$5 \cdot$ Carefully release the bath bomb from the mold and allow it to dry completely for 24–48 hours. Repeat to create the remaining bath bombs.

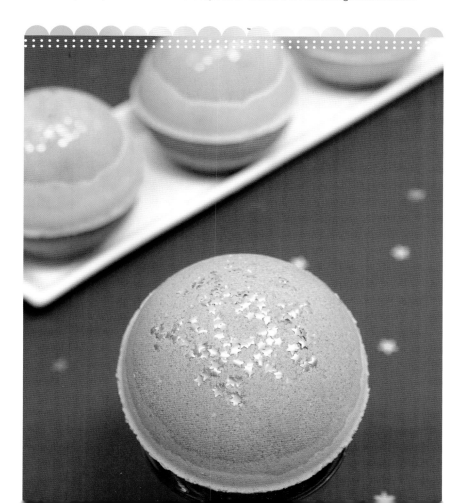

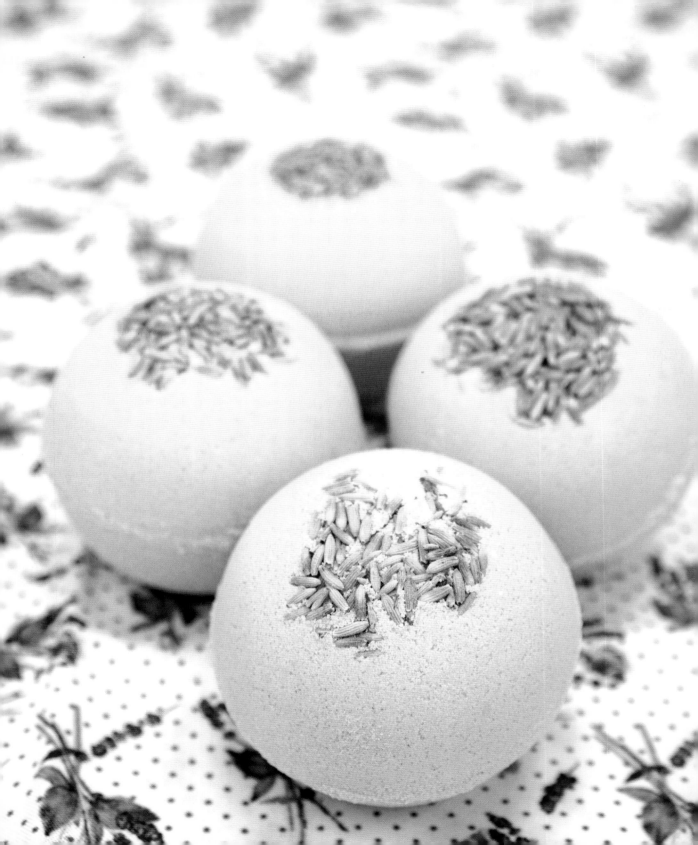

MIND & BODY RELAXATION
BATH BOMBS

Indulging with these relaxing lavender bath bombs is the perfect way to unwind after a busy day! Pink Himalayan salt detoxes skin and soothes tired muscles while the lavender essential oil whisks you away to peace and tranquility.

MAKES

BATH BOMBS

SUPPLIES

1½ cups baking soda

1 tablespoon cream of tartar

1 tablespoon white kaolin clay

⅓ cup pink Himalayan salt, finely ground

2 tablespoons sodium lauryl sulfoacetate (SLSA)

¼ teaspoon purple mica colorant

1½ tablespoons jojoba oil

½ tablespoon polysorbate 80

30 drops lavender essential oil

¾ cup citric acid

Witch hazel, scant amount as needed

Dried lavender buds

2½" round bath bomb mold

MIXING DIRECTIONS

1 · In a large mixing bowl, thoroughly combine the baking soda, cream of tartar, kaolin clay, pink Himalayan salt, SLSA, and purple mica.

2 · In a small container, mix together the jojoba oil, polysorbate 80, and lavender essential oil. Stirring constantly, slowly mix the liquids into the dry ingredients until they are completely combined.

3 · Add the citric acid to the mixture and stir until it is fully incorporated. If the mixture is not quite wet enough to mold, spritz two to three times with a spray bottle of witch hazel and mix well. Repeat as necessary.

MOLDING DIRECTIONS

4 · Place a pinch of lavender buds in the bottom of one half of the mold, and then lightly overfill both halves of the mold with the mixture. Press the halves firmly together.

5 · Carefully release the bath bomb from the mold and allow it to dry completely for 24–48 hours. Repeat to create the remaining bath bombs.

SORE MUSCLE SOAK
BATH BOMBS

Sore, achy muscles? Hit the gym too hard? Too rough at sports practice? These bath bombs are just what you need! The healing combination of emu oil, Epsom salt, and aromatic essential oils helps soothe muscle pain and relax tired joints.

MAKES

10

BATH BOMBS

SUPPLIES

3 cups baking soda

1½ cups Epsom salt, finely ground

2 tablespoons cream of tartar

2 tablespoons sodium lauryl sulfoacetate (SLSA)

1 teaspoon blue mica colorant

1 teaspoon green mica colorant

2 tablespoons sweet almond oil, divided

1 tablespoon emu oil, divided

1 tablespoon polysorbate 80, divided

20 drops peppermint essential oil

10 drops copaiba essential oil

10 drops wintergreen essential oil

6 drops eucalyptus essential oil

1½ cups citric acid, divided

Witch hazel, scant amount as needed

2½" round bath bomb mold

MIXING DIRECTIONS

1 • In a large mixing bowl, thoroughly combine the baking soda, Epsom salt, cream of tartar, and SLSA. Divide the mixture evenly into two medium bowls. Mix the blue mica into one bowl and the green mica into the second bowl.

2 • In a small container, combine 1 tablespoon of the sweet almond oil, ½ tablespoon of the emu oil, ½ tablespoon of the polysorbate 80, 10 drops of the peppermint essential oil, 5 drops of the copaiba essential oil, 5 drops of the wintergreen essential oil, and 3 drops of the eucalyptus essential oil. Stirring constantly, slowly mix the liquids into the blue dry ingredients until they are completely combined. Repeat for the green mixture.

$3 \cdot$ Add ¾ cup of the citric acid to each of the bowls and stir until it is fully incorporated into the mixture. If the mixture is not quite wet enough to mold, spritz two to three times with a spray bottle of witch hazel and mix well. Repeat as necessary.

MOLDING DIRECTIONS

$4 \cdot$ Fill both halves of the mold with the bath bomb mixture in a blue and green striped pattern. Make sure to overfill the mold just a bit. Press the halves firmly together.

$5 \cdot$ Carefully release the bath bomb from the mold and allow it to dry completely for 24–48 hours. Repeat to create the remaining bath bombs.

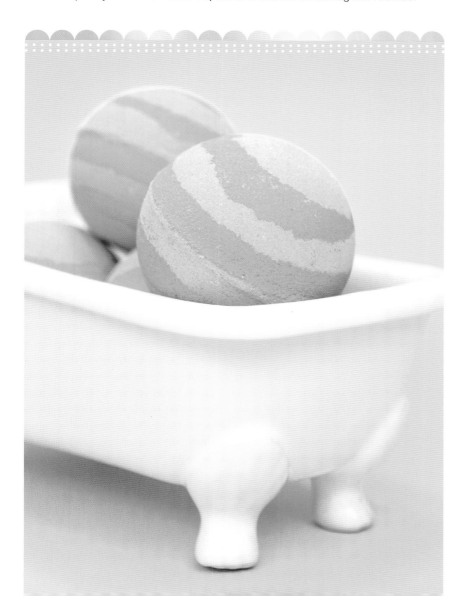

SERENITY
BATH BOMBS

*S*ink into a lavender-tinted pool of serenity beneath a mountain of blissful bubbles. Let the soothing aromas relax your mind and body as the oils hydrate and rejuvenate tired skin.

MAKES

14

BATH BOMBS

SUPPLIES

3 cups baking soda

½ cup Epsom salt, finely ground

2 tablespoons cream of tartar

3 tablespoons sodium lauryl
   sulfoacetate (SLSA)

½ teaspoon purple
   mica colorant

3 tablespoons coconut oil,
   melted and divided

1 tablespoon polysorbate
   80, divided

1 teaspoon cocamidopropyl
   betaine, divided

14 drops lavender essential oil

14 drops Roman chamomile
   essential oil

1½ cups citric acid, divided

Witch hazel, scant
   amount as needed

2″ round bath bomb mold

Chopstick or similar item

MIXING DIRECTIONS

1 · In a large mixing bowl, thoroughly combine the baking soda, Epsom salt, cream of tartar, and SLSA. Divide the mixture evenly into two medium bowls. Stir the purple mica into one bowl and leave the second bowl uncolored.

2 · In a small container, combine 1½ tablespoons of the melted coconut oil, ½ tablespoon of the polysorbate 80, ½ teaspoon of the cocamido-propyl betaine, and the lavender essential oil. Stirring constantly, slowly mix the liquids into the purple dry ingredients until they are completely combined.

3 · In another small container, combine the remaining coconut oil, poly-sorbate 80, and cocamidopropyl betaine with the Roman chamomile essential oil. Stirring constantly, slowly mix the liquids into the white dry ingredients until they are completely combined.

4 · Add ¾ cup of the citric acid to each of the bowls and stir until it is fully incorporated into the mixture. If the mixture is not quite wet enough to mold, spritz two to three times with a spray bottle of witch hazel and mix well. Repeat as necessary.

MOLDING DIRECTIONS

5 · Fill both halves of the mold with alternating areas of white and purple. Use a chopstick to swirl the colors inside each half of the mold. Make sure to overfill both sides of the mold just a bit. Press the halves firmly together.

6 · Carefully release the bath bomb from the mold and allow it to dry completely for 24–48 hours. Repeat to create the remaining bath bombs.

COUGH & COLD
SHOWER STEAMERS

Breathe easier when you're under the weather with natural relief from these shower steamers! Place one in the corner of your shower and take in the airway-opening and antibacterial benefits of peppermint, eucalyptus, and tea tree oils.

MAKES

10

BATH BOMBS

SUPPLIES

3 cups baking soda

2 tablespoons cream of tartar

½ teaspoon blue mica colorant

2 tablespoons sweet almond oil

1 teaspoon polysorbate 80

25 drops peppermint essential oil

15 drops eucalyptus essential oil

10 drops of tea tree oil

½ teaspoon water

¾ cup citric acid

Witch hazel, scant amount as needed

Hard plastic puck mold

MIXING DIRECTIONS

1 · In a large mixing bowl, thoroughly combine the baking soda, cream of tartar, and blue mica.

2 · In a small container, mix together the sweet almond oil, polysorbate 80, peppermint essential oil, eucalyptus essential oil, tea tree essential oil, and water. Stirring constantly, slowly mix the liquids into the dry ingredients until they are completely combined.

3 · Add the citric acid to the mixture and stir until it is fully incorporated. If the mixture is not quite wet enough to mold, spritz two to three times with a spray bottle of witch hazel and mix well. Repeat as necessary.

MOLDING DIRECTIONS

4 · Press the bath bomb mixture firmly into the mold using your thumb and the palm of your hand to apply pressure. Fill the mold to the top until it is packed completely full.

5 · Carefully release the bath bomb from the mold and allow it to dry completely for 24–48 hours. Repeat to create the remaining bath bombs.

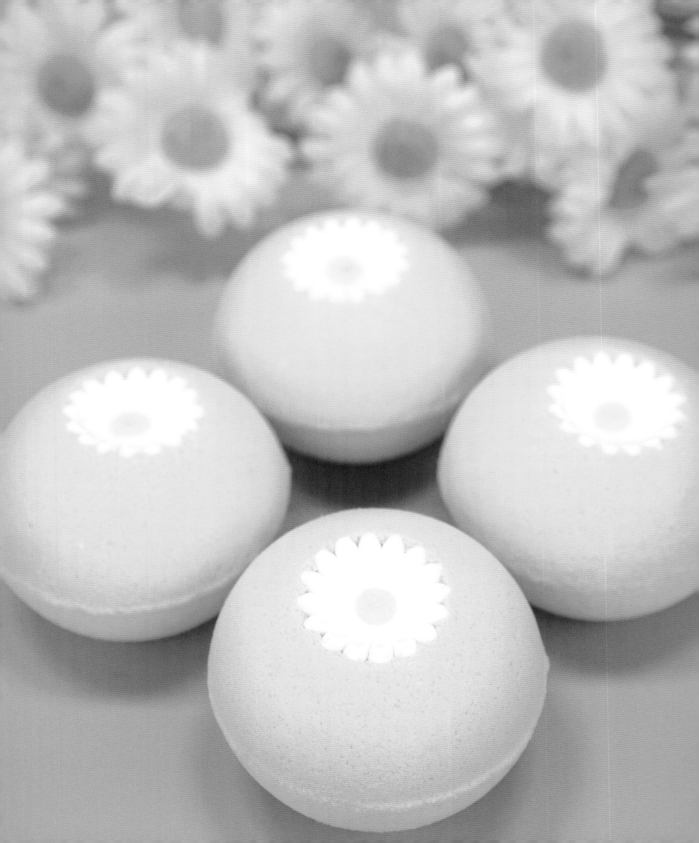

CHAMOMILE BEDTIME
BATH BOMBS

Chamomile has long been known for its relaxing and sleep-inducing properties, making it the perfect addition to these calming bedtime bath bombs. A gentle yellow color sets a calming, pleasant mood to ease you into sleep.

MAKES

5

BATH BOMBS

SUPPLIES

1½ cups baking soda

½ cup Epsom salt, finely ground

1 tablespoon cream of tartar

1 tablespoon white kaolin clay

¼ cup cornstarch

1½ tablespoons sodium lauryl sulfoacetate (SLSA)

½ teaspoon yellow mica colorant

1 tablespoon fractionated coconut oil

½ tablespoon polysorbate 80

20 drops Roman chamomile essential oil

10 drops ylang-ylang essential oil

½ teaspoon water

¾ cup citric acid

Witch hazel, scant amount as needed

8 white candy flowers

2½" round bath bomb mold

MIXING DIRECTIONS

1 · In a large mixing bowl, thoroughly combine the baking soda, Epsom salt, cream of tartar, kaolin clay, cornstarch, SLSA, and yellow mica.

2 · In a small container, mix together the fractionated coconut oil, polysorbate 80, Roman chamomile essential oil, ylang-ylang essential oil, and water. Stirring constantly, slowly mix the liquids into the dry ingredients until they are completely combined.

3 · Add the citric acid to the mixture and stir until it is fully incorporated. If the mixture is not quite wet enough to mold, spritz two to three times with a spray bottle of witch hazel and mix well. Repeat as necessary.

MOLDING DIRECTIONS

4 · Place a candy flower at the bottom of one half of the mold, then lightly overfill both halves of the mold with the mixture. Press the halves firmly together.

5 · Carefully release the bath bomb from the mold and allow it to dry completely for 24–48 hours. Repeat to create the remaining bath bombs.

LAVENDER-OATMEAL
MILK BATH

Soften, smooth, and revitalize dry skin with a refreshing milk bath. This luxurious spa-like treatment will infuse your skin with hydration and can help heal skin conditions, such as eczema, psoriasis, and poison oak/ivy.

MAKES

1

MILK BATH

SUPPLIES

½ cup milk powder

½ cup colloidal oats

¼ cup baking soda

6 drops lavender essential oil

Lavender buds

Storage container

MIXING DIRECTIONS

1 · In a small mixing bowl, thoroughly combine the milk powder, colloidal oats, baking soda, and lavender essential oil.

2 · Use immediately or package in an air-tight container and top with dried lavender buds.

To use · Add the mixture to your bathtub under warm running water.

HOLIDAY

CELEBRATIONS

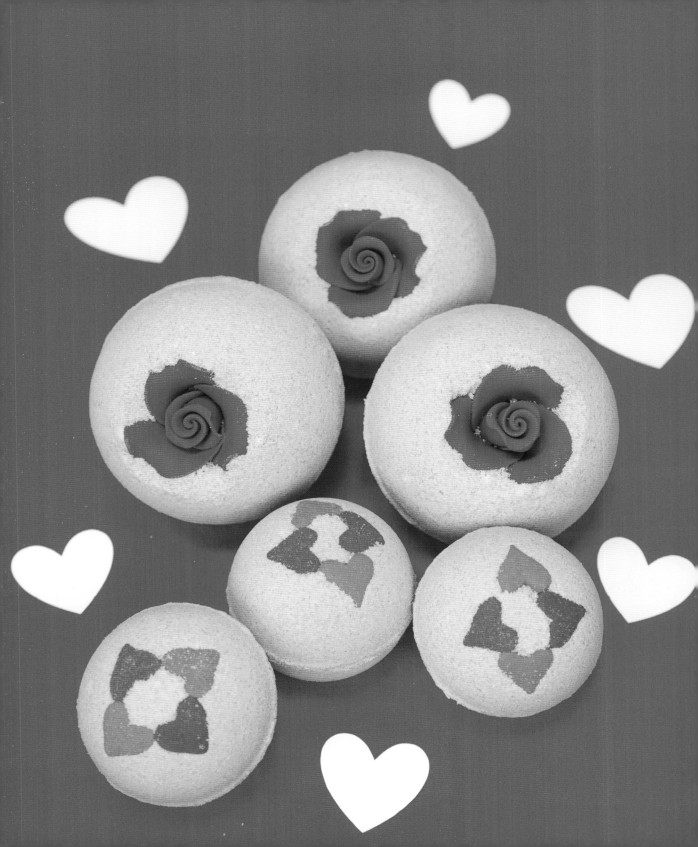

VALENTINE
BATH BOMBS

*W*ish your sweetheart a happy Valentine's Day with these heart- and rose-embellished bath bombs. Infused with the intoxicating fruity-floral aroma of love spell (a popular blend offered with slight variations from different suppliers), these bath bombs are sure to please.

MAKES

BATH BOMBS

SUPPLIES

3 cups baking soda

2 tablespoons cream of tartar

2 tablespoons sodium lauryl sulfoacetate (SLSA)

1 teaspoon pink mica colorant

2 tablespoons sweet almond oil

1 tablespoon polysorbate 80

1 teaspoon love spell fragrance oil

¾ cups citric acid

Witch hazel, scant amount as needed

Red candy icing roses

Extra-large heart sprinkles

2½" round bath bomb mold

MIXING DIRECTIONS

1 · In a large mixing bowl, thoroughly combine the baking soda, cream of tartar, SLSA, and pink mica.

2 · In a small container, mix together the sweet almond oil, polysorbate 80, and love spell fragrance oil. Stirring constantly, slowly mix the liquids into the dry ingredients until they are completely combined.

3 · Add the citric acid to the mixture and stir until it is fully incorporated. If the mixture is not quite wet enough to mold, spritz two to three times with a spray bottle of witch hazel and mix well. Repeat as necessary.

MOLDING DIRECTIONS

4 · Place a candy rose at the bottom of one half of the mold, then lightly overfill both halves of the mold with the mixture. Press the halves firmly together. Alternately, use extra-large heart sprinkles in the bath bombs instead of, or in addition to, the candy roses.

5 · Carefully release the bath bomb from the mold and allow it to dry completely for 24–48 hours. Repeat to create the remaining bath bombs.

LUCKY CHARM
BATH BOMBS

Discover a treasure hidden inside each of these gold-drizzled Irish cream bath bombs! Uncover your lucky charm as you dissolve the bath bomb and fill your tub with a pool of soft green water and shimmery gold fizz.

MAKES

5

BATH BOMBS

SUPPLIES

1½ cups baking soda

½ cup Epsom salt, finely ground

2 tablespoons cream of tartar

½ cup cornstarch

1½ tablespoons sodium lauryl sulfoacetate (SLSA)

½ teaspoon green mica colorant

1 tablespoon apricot kernel oil

½ tablespoon polysorbate 80

½ teaspoon Irish cream fragrance oil

¾ cups citric acid

Witch hazel, scant amount as needed

Mini plastic capsules (approx. 1⅛")

Charms or other small trinkets to fit inside capsules

1 teaspoon gold mica colorant

2 teaspoons isopropyl alcohol

2½" round bath bomb mold

MIXING DIRECTIONS

1 · In a large mixing bowl, thoroughly combine the baking soda, Epsom salt, cream of tartar, cornstarch, SLSA, and green mica.

2 · In a small container, mix together the apricot kernel oil, polysorbate 80, and Irish cream fragrance oil. Stirring constantly, slowly mix the liquids into the dry ingredients until they are completely combined.

3 · Add the citric acid to the mixture and stir until it is fully incorporated. If the mixture is not quite wet enough to mold, spritz two to three times with a spray bottle of witch hazel and mix well. Repeat as necessary.

MOLDING DIRECTIONS

4 · Fill half of the mold with loosely packed bath bomb mixture. Place a charm-filled capsule into the center of the first half of the mold. Fill the second half of the mold, making sure to overfill the mold just a bit. Press the halves firmly together.

5 · Carefully release the bath bomb from the mold and allow it to dry completely for 24–48 hours. Repeat to create the remaining bath bombs.

6 · When the bath bombs are dry, mix together the gold mica and isopropyl alcohol and add gold accents to each bath bomb.

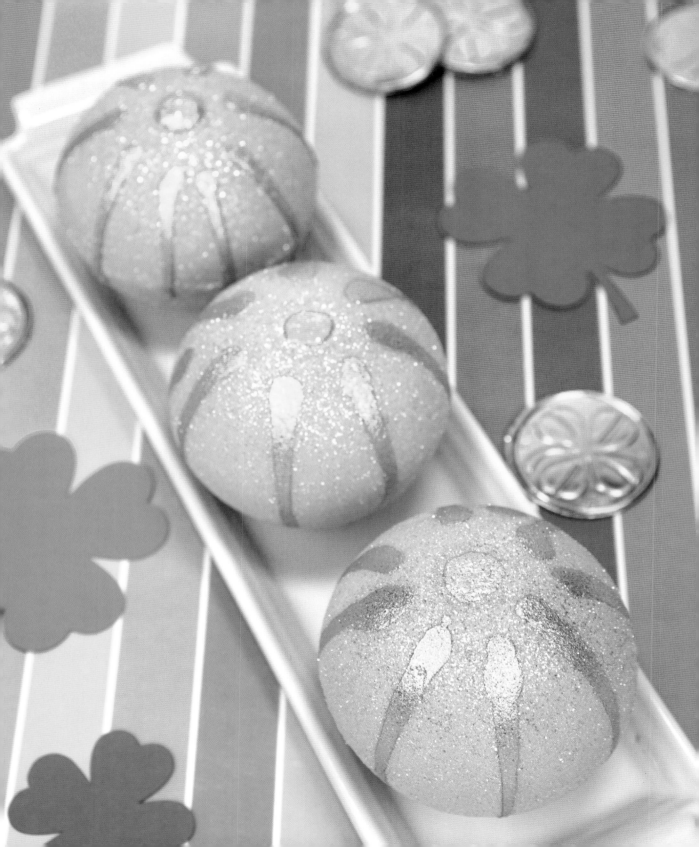

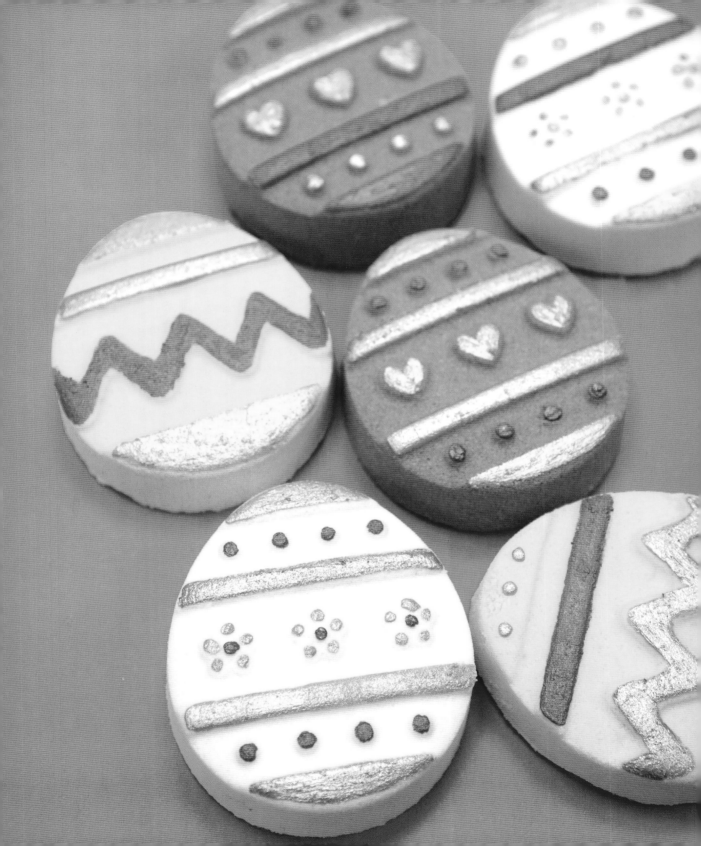

EASTER EGG
BATH BOMBS

Hand-painted bath bombs add color to Easter baskets and the bath. Plus, they offer the moisturizing benefits of shea butter and sweet almond oil. Customize with your favorite colors.

MAKES

18

BATH BOMBS

SUPPLIES

3 cups baking soda

2 tablespoons cream of tartar

2 tablespoons white kaolin clay

2 tablespoons sodium lauryl sulfoacetate (SLSA)

1 teaspoon yellow mica colorant

1 teaspoon purple mica colorant

3 tablespoons sweet almond oil, divided

1½ tablespoons shea butter, melted and divided

1½ tablespoons polysorbate 80, divided

1½ teaspoons marshmallow fragrance oil, divided

1½ cups citric acid, divided

Witch hazel, scant amount as needed

Hard plastic Easter egg mold

Assorted colors of mica for decoration

Isopropyl alcohol

MIXING DIRECTIONS

1 · In a large mixing bowl, thoroughly combine the baking soda, cream of tartar, kaolin clay, and SLSA. Divide the mixture evenly into three medium bowls. Mix the yellow mica into one bowl, the purple into the second bowl, and leave the third bowl uncolored.

2 · In a small container, combine 1 tablespoon of the sweet almond oil, ½ tablespoon of the melted shea butter, ½ tablespoon of the polysorbate 80, and ½ teaspoon of the marshmallow fragrance oil. Stirring constantly, slowly mix the liquids into the yellow dry ingredients until they are completely combined. Repeat this step for each of the different colored bowls.

3 · Add ½ cup of the citric acid to each of the bowls and stir until it is fully incorporated into the mixture. If the mixture is not quite wet enough to mold, spritz two to three times with a spray bottle of witch hazel and mix well. Repeat as necessary.

MOLDING DIRECTIONS

4 · Press the bath bomb mixture firmly into the mold using your thumb and the palm of your hand to apply pressure. Fill the mold to the top until it is packed completely full.

5 · Carefully release the bath bomb from the mold and allow it to dry completely for 24–48 hours. Repeat to create the remaining bath bombs.

6 · When the bath bombs are dry, mix ¼ teaspoon of mica (in color of your choice) with ½ teaspoon of isopropyl alcohol and use a paintbrush to add details to the Easter eggs.

FIRECRACKER
BATH BOMBS

These patriotic firecracker bath bombs are an explosion of fun in your bathtub. Feel your stress lift as you inhale the fresh and fruity aromas of summer and delight in the colorful fizz and bubbles.

MAKES

15

BATH BOMBS

SUPPLIES

3 cups baking soda

½ cup cornstarch

2 tablespoons cream of tartar

2 tablespoons white kaolin clay

2 tablespoons sodium lauryl sulfoacetate (SLSA)

1 teaspoon red mica colorant

1 teaspoon blue mica colorant

3 tablespoons fractionated coconut oil, divided

1½ tablespoons polysorbate 80, divided

½ teaspoon cherry fragrance oil

½ teaspoon coconut fragrance oil

½ teaspoon blue raspberry fragrance oil

1½ cups citric acid, divided

Witch hazel, scant amount as needed

Cyclomethicone liquid, for coating glasses

Floral wire

Disposable plastic cordial glasses

MIXING DIRECTIONS

1 · In a large mixing bowl, thoroughly combine the baking soda, cornstarch, cream of tartar, kaolin clay, and SLSA. Divide the mixture evenly into three medium bowls. Mix the red mica colorant into one bowl, the blue into the second bowl, and leave the third bowl uncolored.

2 · In a small container, combine 1 tablespoon of the fractionated coconut oil, ½ tablespoon of the polysorbate 80, and the cherry fragrance oil. Stirring constantly, slowly mix the liquids into the red dry ingredients until they are completely combined.

3 · In another small container, combine 1 tablespoon of the fractionated coconut oil, ½ tablespoon of the polysorbate 80, and the coconut fragrance oil. Stirring constantly, slowly mix the liquids into the white dry ingredients until they are completely combined.

$4 \cdot$ In a third small container, combine the remaining fractionated coconut oil and polysorbate 80 with the blue raspberry fragrance oil. Stirring constantly, slowly mix the liquids into the blue dry ingredients until they are completely combined.

$5 \cdot$ Add ½ cup of the citric acid to each of the bowls and stir until it is fully incorporated into the mixture. If the mixture is not quite wet enough to mold, spritz two to three times with a spray bottle of witch hazel and mix well. Repeat as necessary.

MOLDING DIRECTIONS

$6 \cdot$ Cut the floral wire into 1½" lengths.

$7 \cdot$ Brush the inside of the cordial glasses with a thin layer of cyclomethicone for easier mold release.

$8 \cdot$ Press the bath bomb mixture firmly into the cordial glasses using your thumb and the palm of your hand to apply pressure. Fill the molds using a red, white, and blue striped pattern until they are packed completely full.

$9 \cdot$ Carefully release the bath bombs from the molds and insert a piece of floral wire into each as the fuse. Allow to dry completely for 24–48 hours.

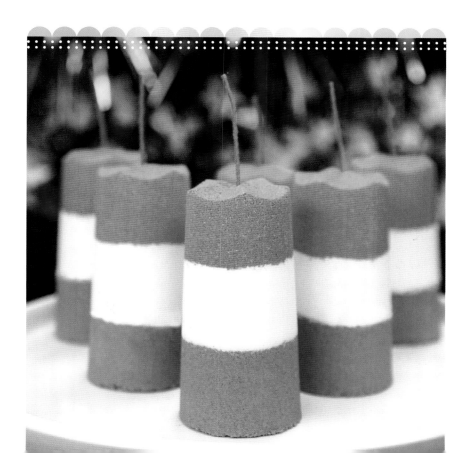

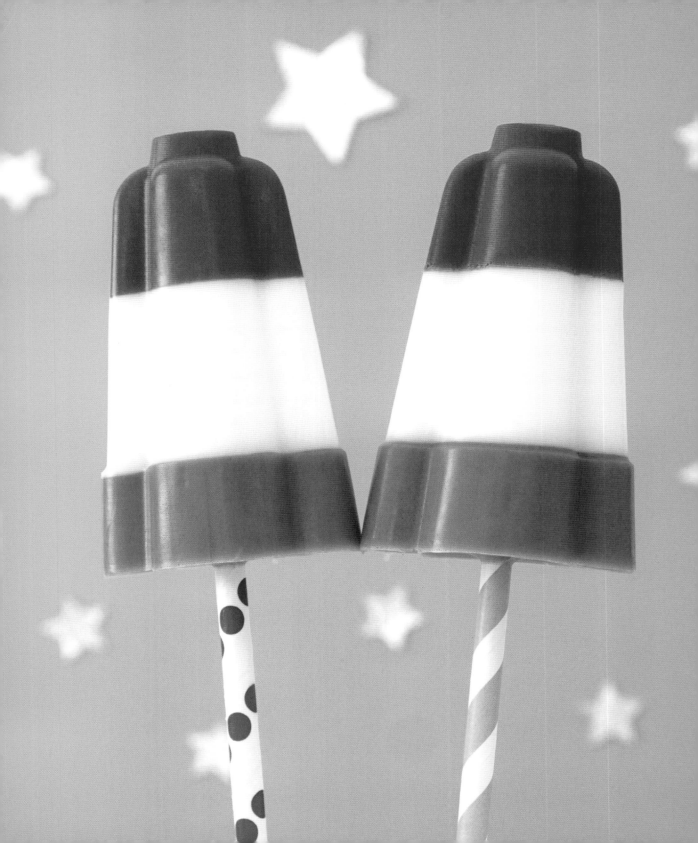

ROCKET POP
SOAPS

These sweetly scented rocket pop soaps look just like the real thing! Lather up in bright summery style with this rich and creamy goat's milk soap that leaves skin feeling fresh and vibrant.

MAKES

SOAPS

SUPPLIES

1 pound goat's milk soap base

Microwave-safe measuring cup

10 drops red soap colorant

15 drops strawberry
  fragrance oil

Silicone rocket pop mold

Isopropyl alcohol, in
  a spray bottle

15 drops coconut fragrance oil

Paper straws

10 drops blue soap colorant

15 drops blueberry fragrance oil

DIRECTIONS

1 · Slice the shea butter soap base into small cubes. Place ¼ pound of the soap cubes into a microwave-safe measuring cup. Melt in the microwave in 30-second increments, stirring well after each session to ensure that the soap is completely melted.

2 · Carefully stir in the red soap colorant and strawberry fragrance oil. Pour the melted soap into the wells of the mold, filling each about ¼ of the way full, and spritz with isopropyl alcohol to remove any air bubbles. Allow to cool for 20 minutes.

3 · Place ½ pound of the soap cubes into a microwave-safe measuring cup and melt in the microwave in 30-second increments. Carefully stir in the coconut fragrance oil. Spritz the red layer of soap with isopropyl alcohol (to help the layers stick together), pour the white soap into the wells of the mold, and spritz with isopropyl alcohol to remove any air bubbles. Gently insert the paper straw into the center of each mold while the white soap layer is still melted. Allow to cool for 30 minutes.

4 · Place ¼ pound of the soap cubes into a microwave-safe measuring cup and melt in the microwave in 30-second increments. Carefully stir in the blue soap colorant and blueberry fragrance oil. Spritz the white layer of soap with isopropyl alcohol, pour the blue soap into the wells of the mold, and spritz with isopropyl alcohol to remove any air bubbles.

5 · Allow the soaps to sit until completely firm (approximately 60–90 minutes) before removing them from the molds.

JACK-O'-LANTERN
BATH BOMBS

It's no trick, all treat with these pumpkin spice-scented jack-o'-lantern bath bombs that pamper skin. Give yourself or little goblins the gift of a refreshing soak in the tub after a long night of trick or treating!

MAKES

15

BATH BOMBS

SUPPLIES

3 cups baking soda

½ cup cornstarch

2 tablespoons cream of tartar

2 tablespoons white kaolin clay

2 tablespoons sodium lauryl sulfoacetate (SLSA)

1 teaspoon purple mica colorant

1½ teaspoons orange mica colorant, divided

1 tablespoon + ½ teaspoon activated charcoal powder, divided

3 tablespoons apricot kernel oil, divided

1½ tablespoons polysorbate 80, divided

1½ teaspoons pumpkin spice fragrance oil, divided

1½ cups citric acid, divided

Witch hazel, scant amount as needed

Hard plastic jack-o'-lantern mold

3 teaspoons isopropyl alcohol, divided

½ teaspoon yellow mica colorant

MIXING DIRECTIONS

1 · In a large mixing bowl, thoroughly combine the baking soda, cornstarch, cream of tartar, kaolin clay, and SLSA. Divide the mixture evenly into three medium bowls. Mix the purple mica into one bowl, 1 teaspoon of the orange mica into the second bowl, and 1 tablespoon of the activated charcoal into the third bowl.

2 · In a small container, combine 1 tablespoon of the apricot kernel oil and ½ tablespoon of the polysorbate 80 with ½ teaspoon of the pumpkin spice fragrance oil. Stirring constantly, slowly mix the liquids into the purple dry ingredients until they are completely combined. Repeat this step for each of the different colored bowls.

3 · Add ½ cup of the citric acid to each of the bowls and stir until it is fully incorporated into the mixture. If the mixture is not quite wet enough to mold, spritz two to three times with a spray bottle of witch hazel and mix well. Repeat as necessary.

MOLDING DIRECTIONS

4 · Press the bath bomb mixture firmly into the mold using your thumb and the palm of your hand to apply pressure. Fill the mold to the top until it is packed completely full.

5 · Carefully release the bath bomb from the mold and allow to dry completely for 24–48 hours. Repeat to create the remaining bath bombs.

6 · When the bath bombs are dry, mix in three separate bowls ½ teaspoon isopropyl alcohol each with the remaining orange mica, the yellow mica, and the remaining activated charcoal powder. Use a paintbrush to apply the facial details to the pumpkins.

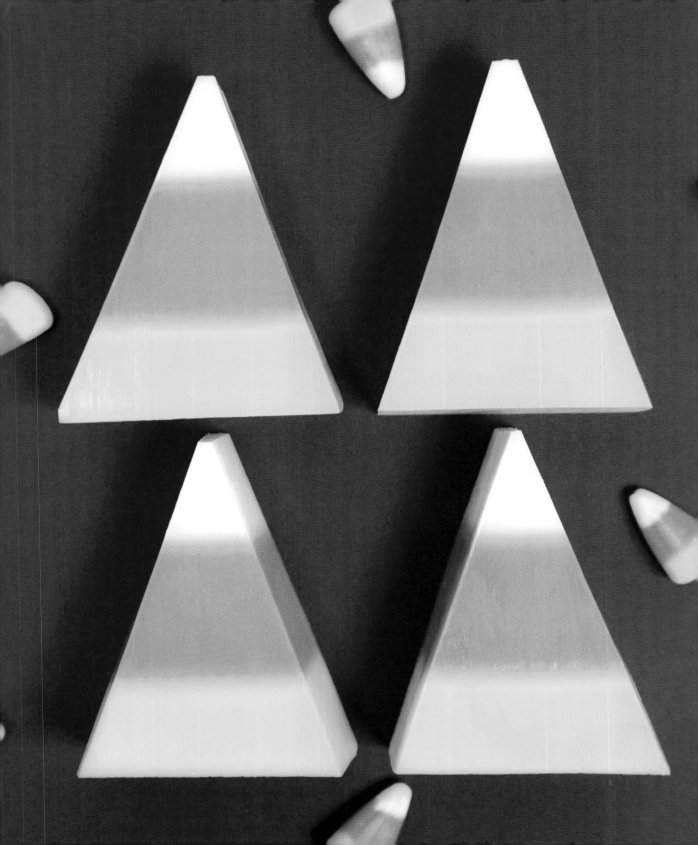

CANDY CORN
SOAPS

These candy corn soaps are a sweet treat in fall, just when dry skin can really start to creep in. Lavish shea butter soap moisturizes and softens while the fragrance will take you back to carefree childhood days.

MAKES

SOAPS

SUPPLIES

1½ pounds shea butter
   soap base, cubed

Microwave-safe measuring cup

10 drops yellow soap colorant

1 teaspoon candy corn
   fragrance oil

24-ounce silicone
   loaf soap mold

Isopropyl alcohol, in
   a spray bottle

10 drops orange soap colorant

DIRECTIONS

1 · Place ½ pound of shea butter soap base cubes into a microwave-safe measuring cup. Melt the soap in the microwave in 30-second increments, stirring well after each session to ensure that it is completely melted.

2 · Carefully stir in 10 drops of yellow soap colorant and ¼ teaspoon candy corn fragrance oil and mix well. Pour the melted soap into the bottom of the soap mold and spritz the top with isopropyl alcohol to remove any air bubbles. Allow to firm for 20 minutes.

3 · Place ½ pound of shea butter soap base cubes into a microwave-safe measuring cup and melt in the microwave in 30-second increments. Add the orange soap colorant and ½ teaspoon of the candy corn fragrance oil. Spritz the top of the yellow layer of soap with isopropyl alcohol (to help the layers stick together), pour the melted orange soap into the mold, and spritz the top with isopropyl alcohol to remove any air bubbles. Allow to firm for 20–30 minutes.

4 · Melt the remaining soap cubes in the microwave in 30-second increments and carefully add the remaining candy corn fragrance oil. Spritz the top of the orange layer with isopropyl alcohol, pour the white soap into the mold, and spritz the top with isopropyl alcohol to remove any air bubbles. Allow to sit undisturbed until completely cooled and firm (2–24 hours depending on temperature and humidity).

5 · Once the loaf of soap is cooled, carefully remove it from the silicone mold. Use a sharp knife to slice the loaf into six individual soaps and trim each soap into a triangle shape to resemble candy corn.

SNOWMAN
BATH BOMBS

*S*nowman bath bombs make great holiday presents! Fill the stockings of friends and family members with the gift of indulgent relaxation. These little snowmen will send them off to bath-time nirvana in a cloud of marshmallow-soft fizz and gentle foaming bubbles.

MAKES

BATH BOMBS

SUPPLIES

3 cups baking soda

1 cup cornstarch

1 cup Epsom salt, finely ground

2 tablespoons cream of tartar

2 tablespoons sodium lauryl sulfoacetate (SLSA)

3 tablespoons fractionated coconut oil

1 teaspoon marshmallow fragrance oil

1½ cups citric acid

Witch hazel, scant amount as needed

Iridescent cosmetic glitter

½ teaspoon activated charcoal powder

½ teaspoon orange mica

2 teaspoons isopropyl alcohol

2½″ round bath bomb mold

MIXING DIRECTIONS

1 · In a large mixing bowl, thoroughly combine the baking soda, cornstarch, Epsom salt, cream of tartar, and SLSA.

2 · In a small container, mix together the fractionated coconut oil and marshmallow fragrance oil. Stirring constantly, slowly mix the liquids into the dry ingredients until they are completely combined.

3 · Add the citric acid to the mixture and stir until it is fully incorporated. If the mixture is not quite wet enough to mold, spritz two to three times with a spray bottle of witch hazel and mix well. Repeat as necessary.

MOLDING DIRECTIONS

4 · Lightly overfill both halves of the mold with the mixture. Press the halves firmly together.

5 · Carefully release the bath bomb from the mold and allow it to dry completely for 24–48 hours. Repeat to create the remaining bath bombs.

6 · When the bath bombs are dry, brush with iridescent cosmetic glitter. Combine 1 teaspoon isopropyl alcohol each with ½ teaspoon activated charcoal powder and orange mica. Use a fine paintbrush to add the snowman's facial details.

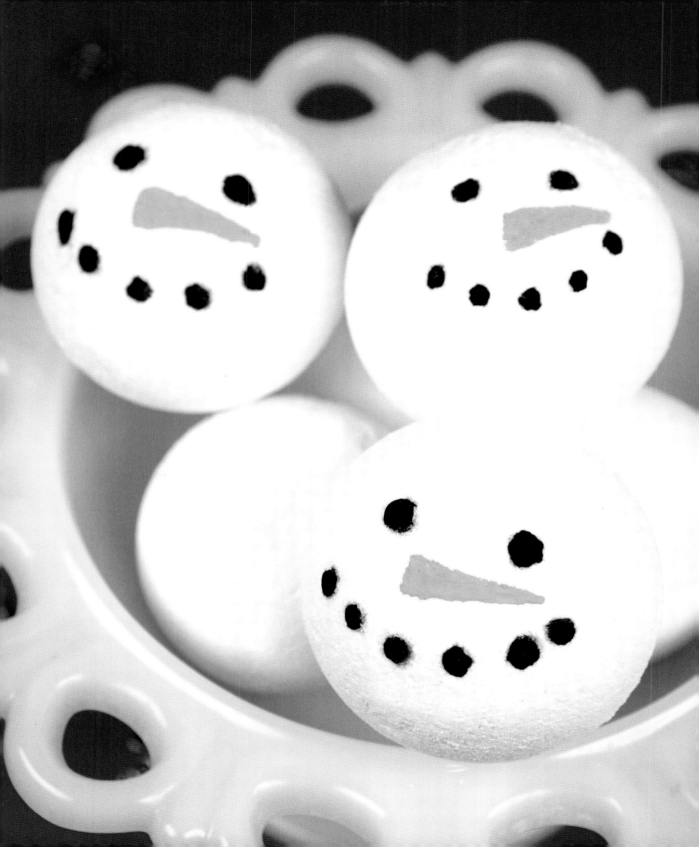

PEPPERMINT BARK
SOAPS

Peppermint oil is the perfect remedy for the busy holiday season! The scent is known for its ability to soothe migraine headaches, calm stomachaches, and alleviate stress. This soap combines the healing benefits of peppermint with the rich aroma of chocolate for a winter treat.

MAKES

8

SOAPS

SUPPLIES

2½ pounds shea butter
   soap base, cubed

Microwave-safe measuring cup

10 drops peppermint
   essential oil, divided

Silicone bar soap mold

Isopropyl alcohol, in
   a spray bottle

20 drops red soap colorant

1 teaspoon chocolate
   mint fragrance oil

15 drops brown soap colorant

8″ square silicone baking pan

DIRECTIONS

1 · Place ¼ pound of shea butter soap base cubes into a microwave-safe measuring cup. Melt the soap in the microwave in 30-second increments, stirring well after each session to ensure that it is completely melted. Add 5 drops of the peppermint essential oil and pour the melted soap into a thin layer at the bottom of 3 or 4 wells of the soap mold. Spritz the top with isopropyl alcohol to remove any air bubbles. Allow to firm for 20 minutes.

2 · Place ¼ pound of the shea butter soap base cubes into a microwave-safe measuring cup and melt the soap in the microwave in 30-second increments. Add the remaining peppermint essential oil and the red soap colorant. Spritz the white layers of soap with isopropyl alcohol (to help the layers stick together) and pour the melted red soap into the mold. Spritz the top with isopropyl alcohol to remove any air bubbles. Allow to sit undisturbed until completely cooled and firm (20–60 minutes depending on temperature and humidity). Unmold and slice into small "peppermint candy" pieces to top the soap.

3 · Place 1½ pounds of shea butter soap base cubes into a microwave-safe measuring cup and melt in the microwave in 30-second increments. Add the chocolate mint fragrance oil and brown soap colorant. Pour the melted soap into the baking pan and spritz the top with isopropyl alcohol to remove any air bubbles. Allow to firm for 30 minutes.

$4 \cdot$ Melt ½ pound of shea butter soap base cubes in the microwave in 30-second increments. Spritz the top of the brown layer with isopropyl alcohol, pour the white soap into the mold, and spritz the top with isopropyl alcohol to remove any air bubbles. Top with the peppermint soap pieces while the white soap is still wet. Push gently on the peppermint pieces to lightly embed them in the surface of the soap.

$5 \cdot$ Allow to sit undisturbed until completely cooled and firm (2–6 hours depending on temperature and humidity).

$6 \cdot$ Once the loaf of soap is cooled, carefully remove it from the silicone mold. Use a sharp knife to slice the loaf into triangular pieces.

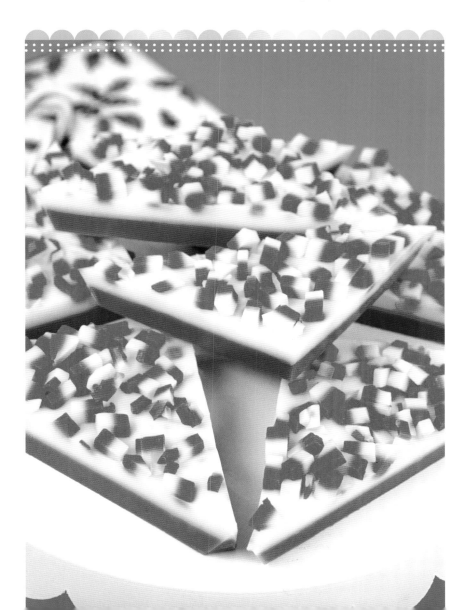

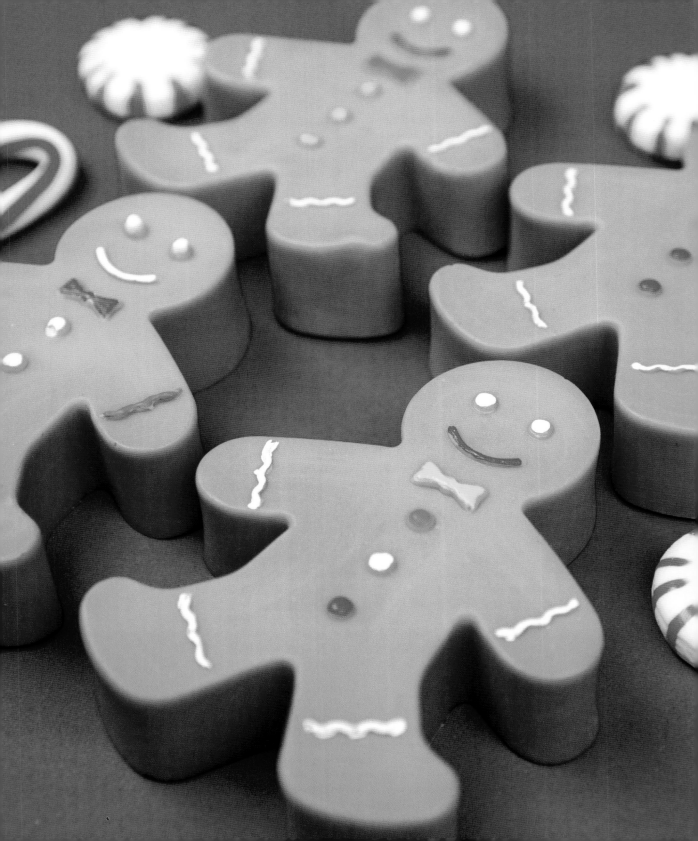

GINGERBREAD MAN
SOAPS

These charming and festive holiday soaps smell just like freshly baked gingerbread cookies, and they're an absolute treat to decorate! Customize each soap using your favorite colors of mica powder paint for super DIY gifts for friends and family.

MAKES

SOAPS

SUPPLIES

1 pound goat's milk soap base

Microwave-safe measuring cup

15 drops brown soap colorant

1 teaspoon gingerbread
   fragrance oil

Isopropyl alcohol, in
   a spray bottle

Assorted colors of
   mica colorant

Silicone gingerbread man mold

DIRECTIONS

1 · Slice the soap base into small cubes and place into a microwave-safe measuring cup. Melt in the microwave in 30-second increments, stirring well after each session to ensure that the soap is completely melted. Carefully stir in the brown soap colorant and gingerbread fragrance oil.

2 · Pour the melted soap into the mold and spritz with isopropyl alcohol to remove any air bubbles.

3 · Allow the soaps to sit undisturbed until completely firm (approximately 60–90 minutes depending on temperature and humidity) before unmolding.

4 · After unmolding, mix ¼ teaspoon mica powder with ½ teaspoon of isopropyl alcohol (for each color) and use a fine paintbrush to paint the gingerbread details.

TROUBLESHOOTING FAQS

$\mathcal{M}$aking bath bombs, soaps, and other bath products can be a tricky process when you're first starting out, but it just takes a bit of practice. Mixtures can be finicky sometimes, and it may take a few tries to discover the recipe that works best for your climate and conditions. If necessary, give your recipe and technique a few tweaks, and you'll be a DIY bath product pro in no time! Here are some of the most common questions:

WHY ARE MY BATH BOMBS SOFT AND CRUMBLY?

Bath bombs that are too soft or crumbly are generally a result of a mixture that was too dry. If the bath bomb mixture doesn't have enough moisture, the bath bombs won't hold together. Increase the amount of oils or add more binder to the mixture.

Conversely, bath bombs can also become soft if there is too much moisture in the mix, so experimentation may be necessary to find the proper ratio of liquid to dry ingredients for your climate. Adding a small amount of kaolin clay or cream of tartar may help to harden overly moist bath bombs.

WHY ARE MY BATH BOMBS CRACKING?

Bath bombs that crack after drying may be a result of too much moisture, either in the mixture or from humidity in the air. Too much moisture can cause a premature fizzing reaction inside the bath bomb that will result in cracking. Bath bombs that have been dried too quickly (in the oven, for example) are also prone to cracking after drying.

WHY WON'T BOTH HALVES OF MY ROUND BATH BOMB STICK TOGETHER?

When bath bombs won't stick together, the culprit is usually one of two issues: (1) The bath bomb mixture is not the proper moldable consistency (too wet or too dry) or (2) the mold has been packed too

tightly and too much pressure was applied. Adjust the mixture's moisture levels and remold using a lighter hand.

WHY DOES MY BATH BOMB HAVE WARTS OR BUMPS ON THE SURFACE?

Warts can occur on the surface of your bath bombs when the wet and dry ingredients were not mixed together well. Clumps of oil, baking soda, or other ingredients can appear as lumps on the surface of your bath bomb. Bumps can also appear if the mixture is too moist. With too much moisture, premature fizzing can occur, releasing carbon dioxide gas from inside the bath bomb and marring the surface.

WHY ARE MY BATH BOMBS EXPANDING OUT OF THE MOLD OR DIFFICULT TO UNMOLD?

Too much moisture can cause bath bombs to activate and expand out of the molds as they are drying. Likewise, this expansion can also make bath bombs difficult to unmold as they grow in size and become stuck inside the mold.

If your mixture is not too wet and the bath bombs are still difficult to unmold, coat the molds with cyclomethicone before molding for easy release. Gently tapping the tops and sides of the mold with a wooden spoon can also help the bath bombs release from the mold.

WHY AREN'T MY BATH BOMBS VERY FIZZY?

There are several reasons why your bath bomb might not be very fizzy. A bath bomb that has been stored in a humid environment can "lose its fizz" over time (due to micro reactions occurring inside the bath bomb).

The recipe itself can also be the issue, depending on your climate and conditions. If you find that your bath bombs aren't very fizzy, you may wish to omit cornstarch and/or SLSA from recipes that include them, as these ingredients can occasionally interfere with the fizzing reaction and slow it down.

WHY ARE MY BATH BOMBS SINKING?

The number one reason that bath bombs sink is because they have been packed too tightly. Try this: just before joining both halves of your round bath bomb mold together, use a chopstick to poke a few small holes into the center of the mixture and create tiny air pockets that will help with buoyancy. Recipes that contain large amounts of heavy oils or butters may also cause bath bombs to sink.

WHAT CAN BE USED TO BIND THE BATH BOMBS IN PLACE OF WITCH HAZEL?

You can use a 50/50 mix of water and isopropyl alcohol to bind the bath bombs instead of witch hazel; however, be aware that binding with alcohol can also lead to crumbly or "dustier" bath bombs.

WHAT IS THE SHELF LIFE OF A BATH BOMB?

Bath bombs are best when they are fresh, making it recommendable to use them within 4 to 6 months. After that time, the bath bombs may lose some of their fizzing potency, and colors and fragrances may begin to fade. Take care to store bath bombs and other bath products out of the reach of young children.

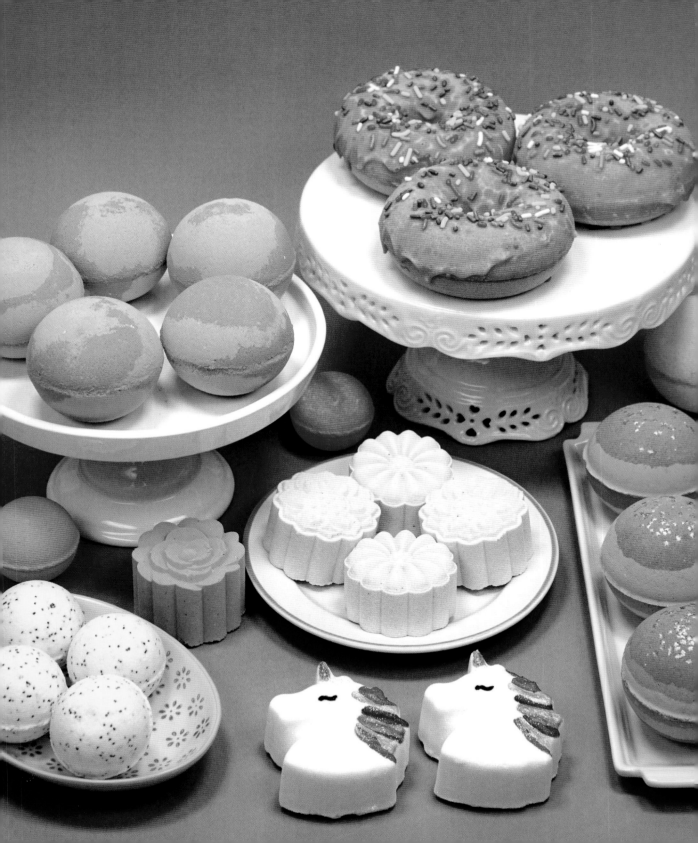